Fernanda C. de Carvalho dos Santos
Henriqueta I. Fernandes
Maria M. S. Ferreira

Nursing Interventions for Child and Adolescent Victims of Abuse

Fernanda C. de Carvalho dos Santos
Henriqueta I. Fernandes
Maria M. S. Ferreira

Nursing Interventions for Child and Adolescent Victims of Abuse

Practices and Behaviours

ScienciaScripts

Imprint

Cover image: www.ingimage.com

This book is a translation from the original published under ISBN 978-613-9-64138-3.

Publisher:
Sciencia Scripts
is a trademark of
Dodo Books Indian Ocean Ltd. and OmniScriptum S.R.L publishing group

120 High Road, East Finchley, London, N2 9ED, United Kingdom
Str. Armeneasca 28/1, office 1, Chisinau MD-2012, Republic of Moldova, Europe
Printed at: see last page
ISBN: 978-620-7-76284-2

To my mum for her constant patience and support, and to my son for his absent moments. With great affection!

ACKNOWLEDGEMENTS

To God, because without him nothing could have been realised.

To Professor Henriqueta Ilda Verganista Martins Fernandes, for the honour of supervising this dissertation and, above all, for her wisdom, trust and teaching throughout this journey.

To Professor Maria Margarida Silva Reis Santos Ferreira, for her availability, critical review and co-supervision of this work.

To Professor Helena Borges Catarino, for making the questionnaire "Child Abuse: Nurses' Practices and Behaviour" available.

To the Executive Board of ACES Grande Porto VII-Gaia for authorising this study.

To the nurses who agreed to take part in this study, making it possible.

To my parents, the best in the world, for their motivation and emotional support.

To my son and my husband for understanding my absence during this period.

Thank you all so much!

CONTENTS

SUMMARY

Abuse perpetrated against children and adolescents is a reality that jeopardises their physical and mental health, compromising their quality of life and well-being both in the present and in the future, as it leaves serious and often irreversible consequences.

The aim of this research was to identify the practices, behaviours, knowledge and training needs of nurses from the ACES Grande Porto VII- Gaia regarding child abuse.

An exploratory, descriptive and correlational study was carried out in which 91 nurses took part. Data was collected between February and March 2013 using a self-completed, anonymous questionnaire. A more detailed analysis of the results regarding the practices and behaviours of the nurses participating in our study towards child/adolescent victims of abuse according to the four sub-scales shows that nurses carry out better practices and behaviours towards child/adolescent victims of abuse in terms of early intervention with children and families at risk (M=3.04). The factor Promoting the child's well-being and safety is the one with the lowest values (M=2.15), contributing little to good practice: The majority of nurses, have come into contact with abused children/adolescents during their professional activity and the most identified situations of danger were neglect, parental/family dysfunction, suspected sexual abuse and physical abuse. The behaviours that could be implemented were referral to social workers, referral to the family doctor and assessing/monitoring the child's behaviour. Of the nurses who reported the situation, the majority did so through the descriptive report.The results highlight that the majority of nurses say they are unaware of the existence of an identification document for families at risk in their unit, as well as a manual of procedures for abuse situations.The majority of nurses do not have specific training in the area of child abuse and expressed great interest in obtaining it. Those who did show an interest in training selected abuse diagnosis, a family intervention programme and the legal framework as their content.

Most nurses emphasised the need to invest in training. This process should be started early in order to prevent abuse.

Keywords: Child; Adolescent; Child Maltreatment; Role of the Nursing Professional

INTRODUCTION

Abuse perpetrated against children and adolescents is a reality that jeopardises their physical and mental health, compromising their quality of life and well-being both in the present and in the future, as it leaves serious and often irreversible consequences.

In scientific, social or clinical practice, the concepts of mistreatment or abuse are often used, and can be considered equivalent to:

> "any form of physical and/or emotional treatment, non-accidental and inappropriate, resulting from dysfunctions and/or deficiencies in interpersonal relationships, in the context of a relationship of dependence (physical, emotional, psychological), trust and power. It can manifest itself through active behaviour (physical, emotional or sexual) or passive behaviour (omission or neglect of care or affection). Through repeated behaviour, they deprive the victim of their rights and freedoms, concretely or potentially affecting their health, development or dignity. Such behaviour should be analysed taking into account the culture and time in which it takes place" (Magalhães, 2010, p.7).

Defining a situation of non-abuse is a complex task, given the many socio-cultural variables (traditions, prejudices, myths associated with many of these practices, particularly corporal punishment).

This idea has been contributed to by international and national studies that demonstrate this problem and, at the same time, highlight the need for an intervention based on scientific knowledge (Calheiros et al., 2011).

Immediate recognition of abuse and rapid intervention by professionals is important for the effective protection of children and adolescents. Its identification should trigger protection and notification actions, in compliance with the provisions of the Law for the Protection of Children and Young People (Oliveira, 2009).Community health services have a fundamental role to play in preventing abuse, as they are the services that have privileged access to families (Soriano Faura, 2009).

The explanatory basis for the occurrence of abuse in children and adolescents is based on the ecological model proposed by Bronfenbrenner (1977). The child/adolescent appears at the centre of a system characterised by a complex network of interrelationships between the microsystem (the inclusive context of the child, abuser and family); the mesosystem (interconnections and processes between the child, abuser and family); the exosystem (interrelationships between the social structure in which the child, abuser and family are inserted) and the macrosystem (beliefs, attitudes, values, ideologies of the social structure).

The choice of the topic "Practices and Behaviours of Primary Health Care Nurses towards Child and Adolescent Victims of Abuse" is related to a professional concern exercised as a nurse at the Support Centre for Children and Young People at Risk (NACJR), the concern revealed by colleagues in dealing with this problem in primary health care (PHC) and the interest in cooperating in improving the nursing care provided to children/adolescents. This activity at the NACJR has allowed us to realise that this is an area that needs more visible intervention, in which there is a clear difficulty for professionals in dealing with these situations. In addition, its social relevance is revealed by the history of child abuse from a salutogenic perspective, which is organised into five periods:

> "Unawareness (until 1946); description of syndromes without identifying them (1946 until 1961); identification (1962 until the mid-1970s); recognition (mid-1970s to mid-1980s) and prevention (since the mid-1980s) (Dias Huertas, cit. by Taveira, 2007, p.11)".

The relevance of the subject is based on the difficulty felt and observed in the context of clinical nursing practice in identifying, notifying and referring situations of child/adolescent abuse, which highlights the need to sensitise nurses to this reality. Nurses are often faced with the dilemma of whether or not they are able to identify, diagnose and intervene in cases of risk and/or danger (Reis, 2009).

The practice and behaviour of professionals in dealing with child and adolescent victims of abuse is closely related to the still obscure visibility of the problem in everyday life. Reflecting on the concepts of the different types of abuse and the ideas associated with them helps to understand how to deal with identifiable cases.

The dissertation "Nurses' Practices and Behaviours towards Child and Adolescent Victims of Abuse" was carried out as part of the Master's Degree in Child Health Nursing and Paediatrics at the Porto School of Nursing.

The starting questions for this research were:

- What are the practices and behaviours of PHC nurses in dealing with abused children and adolescents?
- What knowledge do nurses have about child and adolescent abuse?
- What are nurses' training needs on child abuse?

The aim of this study is to contribute to excellence in nursing care for children and adolescents, with a view to minimising the perpetuation of abuse. Its objectives were:

- To identify nurses' practices with child and adolescent victims of abuse;
- To identify nurses' behaviour towards child and adolescent victims of abuse;
- To identify nurses' knowledge of child abuse;
- Identify nurses' training needs on child abuse.

To this end, we carried out a quantitative, descriptive, exploratory and correlational study with a non-experimental, cross-sectional design. The target population consisted of 91 nurses working in the ACES (Agrupamentos de Centros de Saúde) Grande Porto VII-Gaia who cared for children/adolescents. The five fundamental ethical principles/rights were safeguarded, namely: the right to self-determination, intimacy, anonymity and confidentiality, protection from discomfort and harm, and fair and just treatment (Fortin, 2009).

These ethical principles were a constant concern for us, respecting the rights of the participants involved throughout this research.

The questionnaire "Child Abuse, Practices and Behaviour of Nurses", by Catarino (2007), was used to carry out the research, after the author's permission and consent had been duly requested. The data collected was analysed using descriptive statistics and inferential statistics.

From a structural point of view, this dissertation is divided into three parts:

- The first contextualises ideas about children, adolescence and child abuse. Concepts, typologies, epidemiology are described, risk factors are identified and nurses' practices and behaviours are given particular emphasis. This phase allowed us to go beyond the "simple definition or terminological convention", enabling the "abstract construction that aims to account for the real" (Quivy; Campenhoudt, 2008, p.181).
- The second refers to the methodological framework that led to this research, considering the justification, purpose/objectives, the type of study carried out, the ethical-legal aspects, the description of the collection and statistical treatment of the data.
- The third includes the presentation, analysis and discussion of the results based on national and international research studies that seek to sensitise nurses to this area.

CHAPTER 1

THEORETICAL FRAMEWORK

Scientific research leads to the acquisition of knowledge through a systematic and rigorous process, arising from the researcher's initiative when working on an idea, resulting from observation, personal concern and/or literature review.

Therefore, when the researcher sets out to carry out a research study, it is based on a personal interest stemming from their professional practice, which results in a perceived concern to which they seek an answer (Ribeiro, 2010, p.16).

During the conceptual phase, the researcher "organises their ideas", searches for information and defines a topic or area of research, their conceptualisation "is more than a simple definition or terminological convention. It is an abstract construction that aims to account for reality" (Quivy; Campenhoudt, 2008, p.181). However, for the study to be feasible, its domain must be limited (Vilelas, 2009).

The thematic area selected on the basis of professional concerns is abuse, which is limited to children/adolescents, the practices, behaviours and knowledge of nurses working in PHC and their training needs.

1.1- CHILDREN AND ADOLESCENTS: FROM DEVELOPMENT TO THE FAMILY CONTEXT

The period between childhood and adolescence has long been the subject of study, especially with regard to its implications for human development. The word childhood, the first period of human life, comes from the Latin *infantia,* meaning "inability to speak", and the word infante, from the Latin infante, "one who is unable to speak, without eloquence, very childlike" (Machado, 1997, p. 291).

Throughout time, various scholars have dedicated themselves to the study of human development, understood as "the set of processes through which the particularities of the person and the environment interact to produce constancy and change in the characteristics of the person over the course of their life" (Bronfenbrenner, 1989, p.191).

In this way, we understand child development as an orderly sequence of progressive transformations resulting in an increase in the degree of complexity of the organism (Hochenberry, 2006), with regard to "progressive physical, mental and social growth and development, from birth and throughout childhood" (OE, 2011, p.48).

During this period, children learn through their relationships with others (parents, siblings, friends, teachers...). This learning is multidimensional, simultaneous, unpredictable and continuous, and is also related to life events (affective, communicational).

These assumptions underpin the presentation of a synthesis of the ideas and contributions of different child development scholars:

• Freud (1856 - 1939) contributed to changing the way we think about ourselves, language and culture by emphasising the role of the unconscious in the human mind and considering human behaviour to be the result of a game and an interaction of energies. In the development of the child's personality, he defended the fulfilment of their needs at the different stages of their development, as their neglect has consequences for the formation of their personality (Hochenberry, 2006).

• Erikson (1904 - 1994) further developed Freud's psychosexual theory and its stages, but in opposition to him, he believes that personality is not built solely on sexuality. And in defending the importance of childhood in the development of the child's personality, he considers that it continues to develop beyond the age of five. In his theory, he proposes eight stages of psychosocial development that allow for a healthy transition from childhood to adulthood. At each stage, the child faces and preferably overcomes new challenges or conflicts, which need to be resolved in order to move on to the next stage smoothly and in the time required for each one. Accomplishing them too quickly can have consequences for emotional development and the skills they need to acquire in later life (Hochenberry, 2006).

• Jean Piaget (1896 - 1980). proposed four periods in the evolutionary process of the human species characterised by what the individual can do best: (i) 1st period: sensorimotor (0 to 2 years); (ii) 2nd period: preoperative (2 to 7 years); (iii) 3rd period: concrete operations (7 to 11 or 12 years); (iiii) 4th period: formal operations (11 or 12 years onwards) (Id, 2006).

Generally speaking, all individuals experience these periods in the same sequence. However, the beginning and end of each one may vary depending on the characteristics of the individual's biological structure and the stimuli provided by the environment in which they are inserted. In this way, "the division into these age groups is a reference, not a rigid norm" (Furtado et al., 1999, p.30).

• Lev Vygotsky (1896 - 1934) argued that learning leads to development, since human behaviour functions as a constant overcoming/transformation/suscitation of learning and development throughout its existence. We emphasise that language, as a social instrument of mediation between the Self and the Other, functions as the starting point in the learning/development relationship. In this way, language can be understood as the basis for the entire constitutive process of human subjectivity, because "behind every thought there are desires, needs, interests and emotions, so that understanding what we say depends substantially on our listener's interaction with this affective-volitional basis" (Jobim; Souza, 2001, p. 24).

• From his systematic approach, Skinner (1904 - 1990) sought to understand human behaviour in its relationship with cultural beliefs and practices. He investigated the shaping of behaviour by positive and/or negative reinforcement. He advocated operant conditioning, in which a certain behaviour is more likely to be repeated if it is followed by positive and pleasant reinforcement. This form of conditioning can lead to the behaviour occurring before the response. From this perspective, environmental stimuli play an important role in learning, so children can show relatively stable behavioural changes that are linked to their experiences (Filho, et al, 2009).

- Albert Bandura (1925 - present) believes that children learn by interacting with their environment and observing others. The environment shapes the child's personality and behaviour and the links between people, behaviour and the environment are bidirectional. Thus, children can influence their environment through their behaviour (Fonseca, 2005).
- Urie Bronfenbrenner (1917 - present). views the human being from a global and integrated point of view, with the concept of the person framed within the context of life, environment and surroundings that establish a mutual interaction between them and influence each other (Martins; Szymanski, 2004).

The concept of adolescence comes from the Latin word *"adolescere" and* corresponds to the period of human life that follows childhood, marked by intense conflictual processes and persistent efforts at self-affirmation, the absorption of social values and the development of projects that imply full social integration (Vilela, 2009). It is a process of maturation as attitudes and competences for effective social participation are acquired and adjusted (Id, 2009).

The World Health Organisation (WHO, 2002) considers individuals between the ages of 10 and 19 to be adolescents and divides adolescence into three phases: (i) early, between the ages of 10 and 13; (ii) middle, between the ages of 14 and 15, and (iii) late, between the ages of 16 and 19.

Adolescence is a dynamic process of moving from childhood to adulthood, which is not an easy task "it's a bit as if something very important had been lost and something very important had not yet been found" (Costa, 1998, p.8).

Today's approach to adolescence goes beyond the fact that it is a period of great change. It is important to understand it from the perspective of a period in the life cycle marked by discovery and multiple opportunities arising from different social and cultural contexts. It is therefore important to understand the ideas of some scholars on adolescence:

- Erikson referred to the "crisis of adolescence" as a process of psychosocial transformation characterised by contradictions and ambivalence, with adolescents living in a permanent oscillation between two poles: independence (the need for autonomy) and dependence (the manifest need for protection) (Vilelas, 2009).
- Freud did not identify adolescence as a distinct stage in development, even though he considered it crucial. His perspective favoured the person as having a reservoir of basic biological impulses, identifying the emergence of a certain aspect of human sexuality at each distinct stage of the life cycle. In adolescence, various sexual and aggressive impulses experienced by the individual in the early stages of their development (oral, anal and oedipal) are reactivated in a mature and genital form. Intellectualisation is the defence mechanism adopted by the adolescent to deal with his

emotional revolt, leading him to change the concrete issues of the body to more abstract and emotionless ones. Therefore, the conflicts of puberty are considered normal and necessary for adaptation and the search for a new sense of personality and social role (Senna; Dessen, 2012).

- Piaget said that the adolescent behaviours that cause concern for adults have their origins in the changes in their way of thinking, characteristic of the beginning of this phase. With the development of formal thought, through the assimilation and accommodation of new structures, adolescents reveal their own way of understanding their reality and construct philosophical, ethical and political systems in an attempt to adapt and change the world (Coll et al.,1996,Inhelder, Piaget, 1958-1976, cited by Catarino, 2009). By realising that solutions based on logical reasoning alone are not possible, adolescents reach adulthood by inserting themselves into society (Catarino, 2009).
- Brofenbrenner considered adolescents to be people with their own individual, psychological and biological characteristics, as well as their own way of dealing with their life experiences. They are active subjects, products and producers of their development, which takes place in interaction with their context. This context is defined by a hierarchy of interdependent systems - micro, meso, exo and macrosystem - and is made up of the activities, roles and interpersonal relationships present, for example, in their family, groups of friends, neighbourhood, community, and educational, health, social and political institutions (Bronfenbrenner, 1999).

In adolescence, one can recognise the direct and indirect effects generated by the successive changes and stabilities that occur not only in individual characteristics, but above all in the historical-cultural, social, political and economic transformations attributed to the time in which it is lived (Bronfenbrenner, 1996).

Costa (2002) argues that adolescents coexist in the world in relation to their environment, as interlocutors of a culture in a personal context of realisations in which family, social, political and religious dimensions challenge them to become a person. The author adds that adolescence is a life journey that is particularly influenced by the cultural standards and values of each society.

In order to understand human development in childhood and adolescence, it is necessary to realise which factors interfere with it. These are related to the child/adolescent, the family and society. According to Brazelton (2000), the influences of the internal environment (biological and psychological) and the external environment (social environment) begin to act even before birth and continue throughout life. Therefore, in order for the child/adolescent to have a balanced development, basic needs must be met, with the aim of improving autonomy and the care inherent to well-being (Catarino, 2007).

Many scientific studies point to the importance of early interaction, parent-child relationships and parenting practices. These include studies by Barudy (1998), Bowbly (2002), Brazelton (2000) and Ribeiro (2003).

These authors consider that the affective relationship with the family is one of the cornerstones of the child's/adolescent's development, making its presence synonymous with well-being and protection against loneliness, suffering and anguish. According to Ribeiro (2003), specific parental behaviours and attitudes influence the common development of the child/adolescent and the family itself.

The family, being a complex structure, is made up of elements whose union derives from blood and emotional ties and is the natural context in which to be born and grow up. At the same time, it should generate love and, in some circumstances, it can also cause suffering (Relvas, 2000). This makes it possible to say that the family is both a whole and parts, with the sum of the parts being greater than the whole.

Carneiro (1997) argues that the family is not a simple natural phenomenon, it is a social institution that varies throughout history and can have different forms and functions at the same time, place and according to the social group in which it is inserted.

The current view of the family is that it is a dynamic system, changing internally and in continuous relationship with the outside world. This concept allows it to be perceived as a unique and complex system, where relationships and interactions of reciprocity and interdependence are established, as well as having evolutionary and contextual dimensions (Relvas, 2000).

According to Ferreira (2002), a family's traditional values depend on the culture in which it is located. This is why the child/adolescent assimilates or interprets them in a particular and variable way, depending on the developmental stage they are at. The health of children/adolescents is achieved by prioritising their growth and development within the family context (Sousa; Carvalho, 1990; Ferreira, 2002).

According to Gimeno (2001), the basic functions of the family are economic, reproductive and personal development, with an emphasis on individualisation, self-realisation and an egalitarian role model. In this way, it encompasses physical and emotional health, protection, affection for all its members and active integration into the social environment.

The role of the family fulfils two types of objectives: an internal one, the psychosocial protection of its members, and an external one, the accommodation and transmission of a culture. The home is therefore the right place for the individual to develop fully, whether or not they can benefit from the family atmosphere (Reis, 2009).

The family as a social system has functional prerequisites such as the ability to adapt, realise goals, integrate, maintain standards and control tensions. In this way, it constitutes a cosy environment for the child/adolescent and is capable of guaranteeing their full security. The bond between the different family members is a central element in the process of socialisation and emotional balance (Ambrósio, 1992).

The family unit is responsible for providing the protection and socialisation measures that lead to the harmonious human development of the child/adolescent and the quality of the care they receive. In this sense, the role of the family is a "series of activities and relationships expected of a person who occupies a certain position in society and of others in relation to that person" (Bronfenbrenner, 2002, p.68). This role can be provider, homemaker, caregiver, socialising, therapeutic, recreational and parental (Id, 2002).

The effective fulfilment of the parental role implies the existence of a stable and coherent environment that allows the child/adolescent to feel truly loved and loving. In this sense, relationships in the family environment must involve affection that allows them to assume feelings of security and belonging.

On the other hand, parental failure to fulfil needs generates feelings of rejection with serious consequences for the child/adolescent (Catarino, 2009).

In this way, it can be seen that there are factors that enhance the tension of performing the family role, such as the inability to define the situation, the lack of knowledge and consensus, role conflict, role saturation and power (Hanson, 2005). In this context, power is understood as "the ultimate ability or capacity of actors to produce or cause (expected) results or effects, particularly in the behaviour of another or in the results of another" (Szinovacz, 1987, p.652).

Family leadership stems from the fact that it is a "social system" that has to "fulfil functions and achieve goals", which is why it "needs internal organisation and a distribution of roles" (Gimeno, 2001, p.90). The imbalance between these two aspects gives rise to family conflict. However, despite its existence, the family maintains its uniqueness and its role as a determining factor in the development of sociability, affectivity and the physical well-being of its members (Relvas, 2000).

The absence of a family or even belonging to an unbalanced family jeopardises the integral development of children/adolescents and can potentiate the appearance of risk situations, namely alcohol and tobacco consumption and teenage pregnancy. When children/adolescents have a relationship of well-being, education, work and community life, they are more likely to become sociable and adapt to the stipulated social norms (Reis, 2009).

In the family environment, children/adolescents are more likely to find the conditions that are essential for their development: love, protection, security and heterogeneity (Reis, 2009). According to Sarmento (2005, p.16) "the family nucleus is a problematic and critical place, where both affection and dysfunctionality can be found, both welcome and abuse"

Once the importance of the family in the development of children/adolescents is recognised, the lack of it can affect their relationship with others, due to the relational difficulties that have marked their journey. The impairment of their identity process interferes with their psychological development and can be reflected in their way of relating and in their perception and understanding of those around them (Fonseca, 2002).

The family plays an important role in the overall development of the child/adolescent and in their process of integration into society, and consequently in preventing situations of abuse. Most scholars on the subject are now unanimous in considering changes in family functioning as one of the main causes of behavioural disorders, including violence in the family (Fonseca, 2002; Sarmento, 2005; Magalhães, 2010). In other words, there are no children in danger without families in danger, which once again raises the need for protection and the responsibility of nurses as promoters of healthy development, as the family is the main social group "at risk" when it comes to the phenomenon of violence (Reis, 2009).

In an attached child/adolescent, the trust they have in themselves and in the Other facilitates a warm and trusting interpersonal relationship, whereas those who are insecurely attached have negative expectations of themselves and of the trust they place in the Other (Bowlby, 1981).

Many of these children/adolescents continue to be ignored victims because the trauma or psychological damage they have suffered is not understood. On an emotional level, according to Burrington, it is common for them to "manifest reactions of avoidance, fear, aggression, guilt, shame, sadness, anxiety, insecurity and confusion" (1999, p.102, cited by Machado; Gonçalves, 2002). In addition, there are changes in their self-concept, relationships, goals and life projects.

The abused child/adolescent runs the risk of developing negative global models. Negative expectations about themselves and the Other also have a negative influence on their ability to interact properly, and they are not prepared to develop positive and successful relationships (Mueller; Silverman, 1989; Magalhães, 2010).

From the point of view of parental functions, it is the parents' responsibility to provide the protection and socialisation measures that are theirs by right, so the quality of the care the child receives is their responsibility (Ribeiro, 2003), as their role is to:

> "Interacting in accordance with the responsibility of parenthood; internalising the expectations held by family members, friends and society regarding the appropriate or inappropriate behaviour of the role of parent, expressing these expectations in the form of behaviour, values; above all in relation to promoting the optimal growth and development of a dependent child" (OE, 2011, p.66).

1.2- CHILD/ADOLESCENT ABUSE: FROM HISTORY TO THE PRESENT DAY

Abuse is not a new phenomenon, nor is it exclusive to Westernised societies. The social and cultural figure of childhood and the forms of child/adolescent abuse have been constructed differently throughout different socio-historical eras (Magalhães, 2010).

In the past, many practices of abuse and domestic violence were socially accepted, and today they are considered to disrespect human rights. These historical roots can contribute to our current understanding of this phenomenon. In the present, cultural aspects linked to violence against children/adolescents and the historical social representation of childhood intersect (Magalhães, 2010).

In ancient times, infanticide was practised in all Eastern and Western cultures until the 4th century AD. Its practice was based, among other things, on the elimination of newborns with congenital malformations, premature babies and in response to religious beliefs (Canha, 2003).

In this sense, the following stand out:

- In Roman society, it was customary to immolate first-born children when the king's life was in danger. Aristotle and Plato defended this practice, but drew teachers' attention to the importance of teaching without punishment (Reis, 2009).
- In Ancient Rome, parents had the right to sell, kill or choose whether or not to let their

children live. The ancient Greeks practised infanticide and the abandonment of newborns with malformations. There are also stories of child abuse in the Bible (Magalhães, 2005).

These practices only took on the dimension of mistreatment over the centuries and this slow change in perspective and feelings may be associated with a change in the concept of childhood as a fundamental stage of life (Magalhães, 2005). From the Middle Ages to the Renaissance, children were devalued and compared to the elderly and/or alcoholics (Soares, 1997).

Between the 14th and 17th centuries, children, who until then had been handed over to nannies or institutions, became part of the family's emotional life. A time when
A number of institutions emerged with the aim of protecting and educating them, recommending moderation in the practice of physical punishment (Magalhães, 2010). We can say that until the 17th century, children played a very small role in the family and in society, with the distinction between children and adults being almost non-existent, as they shared work, entertainment and even clothing. Likewise, there was little concern about chronological age, many were unaware of their age and exact birth records were rare (Canha, 2003).

From the end of the 17th century to the beginning of the 18th century, the rate of infanticide and child abandonment was very high, which is why asylums or orphanages specialised in taking in minors began to spring up in various European countries (Magalhães, 2010). Many children died and were buried without the knowledge of others, especially those born of extramarital relationships. In the most disadvantaged families, they were also looked down upon, and from an early age, they were integrated into the world of work, being considered a "miniature adult" who contributed to the family's livelihood. It was in this historical and social context that mistreatment at work came to exist in a more or less camouflaged form, a situation that continued for a long time (Canha, 2003, p.7).

In the 18th century there was a significant improvement in the sanitary conditions of the population, and as a result infanticide and infant mortality decreased. Also, during that century and the beginning of the next, many children were interned in institutions as a protective measure. This was more in the interests of the community than the child itself, but it was considered a lesser evil when compared to infanticide (Id, 2003).

At this time, Jean-Jacque Rousseau considered children to have their own values and potential. His ideas spread and influenced educators, doctors and teachers (Magalhães, 2005).

The French Revolution (1789 - 1799) enabled the liberation of the oppressed: the poor, the insane and children. This led to protection laws and the universalisation of schools and protective institutions. From then on, childhood began to be viewed differently and was recognised as a specific stage of life that required special care (Id, 2010).

In the 19th century, in 1857, the laws stemming from the French Revolution were reinforced. However, the Industrial Revolution (1760-1840) brought new manufacturing processes, creating labour conditions for the exploitation of children/adolescents (Magalhães, 2010). In this century, Taveira (2007, p.16) highlighted four events that had an impact on abuse: the scientific study of real cases, the creation of the first children's hospitals, the increase in remuneration for child labour and the appearance of the first societies dedicated to "preventing cruelty inflicted on children". The same author argues that the increase in social control and the generalisation of child abandonment were helped, for example, by the concealment of signs of physical violence during medical consultations by parents/guardians and the interest in studying these situations in depth.

The determinants of social awareness were the following events:

- The *Child Welfare Movement* in the United States of America in 1825, the result of cultural changes that led to the emergence of the New York Society for the Reform of Juvenile Delinquents, creating a space for vagrant and/or abandoned and/or abused children (Taveira, 2007);
- The "*Society for Prevention of Cruelty to Children" was* founded in New York to prevent child violence, a movement that arose from the publicising of a case that shocked society:

> "A four-year-old girl (...) was beaten and spent most of the day tied to the foot of her bed with chains (...) neighbours reported the case. However, as child abuse was not considered an offence, the case was referred to the Animal Protection Society (...) on the grounds that this child belonged to this level of the zoological scale (Gallardo, 1994, p.20);

- The scientific description of the syndrome of the maltreated child, in the work *"Étude médico-légale sur les sevices et mauvais traitements exercés sur les enfants*", written in 1852, by Toulmuche, a French coroner (Magalhães, 2010, p.15);
- The report produced in 1860 by Ambroise Tardieu, a professor of forensic medicine in Paris, in which he described 32 cases of abused children, pointing out the injuries suffered, family problems and the contrast between clinical data and parental justifications. Approximately 30 years after its publication, a law was passed to protect abused children (Taveira, 2007);
- The appearance of the first paediatric hospitals in Paris and London (Id, 2007);
- The creation of UNICEF (United Nations Children's Fund) in 1947, in the post-World War II period, which emphasised the notion of well-being (Taveira, 2007).

Reis (2009) reinforces the idea that the emergence of new social institutions in the United States increased public awareness of abused children, and legislative measures were enacted to minimise these situations.

During the 20th century, there were social movements that led to legal and scientific changes, among which we highlight the following:

- The manifestation of workers and educators specialising in abused children, however, the real awareness on the part of these professionals only gained relevance in the early 1960s (Magalhães, 2005);
- The historical tradition of violence against children and adolescents and the socio-cultural tolerance of child abuse have contributed to its late recognition as a serious social problem that has victimised and continues to victimise countless children and young people (Canha, 2003).

The legal changes resulting from these movements led to the approval of:

- Universal Declaration of Human Rights in 1948;

• Declaration of the Rights of the Child in 1959 by the United Nations Organisation (UNO);

• The "European Charter on the Rights of the Child" in 1992, approved by the European Parliament, which, in addition to establishing the rights of the child in European countries, asked member states to appoint a defender of these rights (Magalhães, 2005).

Advances in the scientific field were made with the emergence of the first conceptual definition of maltreatment. From 1965 onwards, the term "maltreated child syndrome" came to include physically, emotionally, sexually, abandoned and nutritionally abused children (Kempe; Kempe, 1985). Abuse of minors has acquired a new and broad dimension, which includes active and passive forms, emotional and physical aspects, family and extra-family contexts and physical and psychological needs. Together, these aspects have made it possible to identify possible consequences and transgenerational repercussions (Magalhães, 2005).

In Portugal, the study of child abuse began in the 1980s, more specifically in 1985, when the Centre for the Study of Abused Children at the Coimbra Paediatric Hospital was set up (Canha, 2003). In 1989, Fausto carried out an investigation into child abuse in the cities of Lisbon and Porto, which came to be considered a pilot study and served as the basis for later investigations at a national level.

The Convention on the Rights of the Child (CRC) was approved by the General Assembly and ratified in Portugal on 21 September 1990, constituting a historic milestone. This convention reinforces the notion that all children need special care, and that parents are responsible for their child's protection, education, health and well-being (Magalhães, 2005).

Despite having ratified the CRC, it is still far from achieving the goal of all children having the opportunities and rights to enjoy healthy overall development. This is due to the lack of resources, budgets and people involved in this process (Magalhães, 2010). According to the Institute for Child Support (IAC), Portugal is considered to be a country where the existing means have not yet reached the desired targets so that we can get closer to the "best health indicators achieved in the region of the world where we live - the European Union" (IAC, 2002, p.9).

With regard to this Convention, Martins (2004, p.75) states that it opened up "new and more complex understandings of the concrete ways in which the right to protection can be exercised", in relation to the provision of social, cultural, economic and civil rights for children/adolescents, driving their absolute development.

The CRC recognises the child's right to enjoy the healthiest possible state and to benefit from medical and re-education services (IAC, 2002). The creation of the National Health System was also a milestone in the realisation of these rights. However, there are still behaviours created by social circumstances exogenous to this system that lead to the subsistence of child labour, child abuse in the family context and rates of school dropout and absenteeism. The right to health is an essential right provided for in the Constitution of the Portuguese Republic, i.e. all citizens have the right to promote and defend the protection of health, whether their own or that of others, particularly children/adolescents in families at risk (Peixoto, 2007).

According to Azevedo and Maia (2006), the educational models practised by parents and educators in Portugal are linked to certain cultural and social stigmas instilled in the past:

- It is a traditionalist organisation where education is carried out with discipline, using "processes that are as obsolete as they are cruel";
- the "supposedly" modern world where roles and responsibilities are unknown, promoting a transposition of the "hierarchical family relationship, not providing children with a firm and coherent model" (Id, 2006, p.22);
- and another model in which educators "fall victim to their own ignorance, history or life contexts" and renounce their "responsibilities, disregarding or ignoring, intentionally or not" their role as educators (Id, 2006, p.22).

Children/adolescents who come from these models are considered to be minors who are victims of abandonment, physical and/or psychological violence or even sexual abuse, resulting from reprehensible procedures that jeopardise their safety, health, moral and educational training (Peixoto, 2007). Therefore, there is a need to defend them by intervening directly or indirectly in family and educational contexts.

The adaptation of Portuguese legislation to the international reality in the scientific, cultural and social areas favoured the creation:

- of the IAC in 1983, with the primary objective of defending the rights of the child, enshrined in the United Nations Convention on the Rights of the Child, approved on 20 November 1989;
- In 1991, the Comissão de Proteção de Menores (CPM - Commissions for the Protection of Minors) were created, which are unofficial institutions that operate within local councils and include professionals from various fields, such as education, health, social action and others. These committees, according to Almeida et al. (2001, p.31-32), "have the power to intervene with individuals up to the age of 18 (...) as long as they are involved in situations of abuse or with those whose health, safety or education is at risk". Later, in 1999, the CPM were renamed Commissions for the Protection of Children and Young People in Danger (CPCJ) and played a fundamental role in society. As official non-judicial bodies that include various members of the community, they play a fundamental role in preventing and intervening in situations of risk for families of children and young people (Martins, 2004). Today, CPCJs are scattered throughout the country and develop individualised forms of protection, playing an important role in the system for protecting children and adolescents in danger. As official non-judicial institutions with functional autonomy, they represent the duty and responsibility to promote, defend and respect their rights (CNPCJR, 2011);
- of the Interministerial Commission between the Ministries of Justice and Solidarity and Social Security in 1998, which defined the concept of children at risk: all those whose behaviour jeopardises their own growth and/or whose parents do not provide the necessary care (Magalhães, 2005).

From a legal point of view, in 1999 we highlight the Law for the Protection of Children and Young People in Danger, which only came into force in 2001 and whose purpose is to promote the rights and protect children and young people in danger, in order to guarantee their well-being and integral development (Magalhães, 2005). This law allows anyone who is aware of situations that jeopardise the life, physical or psychological integrity or freedom of a child/young person to report them to the bodies with competence in this area, namely the CPCJ and/or the Judicial Authorities. As Magalhães (2005) states, the main objective of the CPCJ is to remove the danger in which minors find themselves and they are defined by members of the Public Prosecutor's Office, so that efficient articulation and coordination with the various players at community, administrative and judicial level are safeguarded (Epifânio; Pedroso, Cit. by Martins, 2004).

Azevedo and Maia admit that the situations of children/adolescents at risk are related to a complex social reality, "where multiple and varied factors interact". And this "remains an open question that requires an interdisciplinary and systemic approach" capable of providing a global view of the whole problem (2006, p.45).

Armando Leandro (cited by Azevedo; Maia, 2006, p.71) considers that the use of punishments and rigid education in Portugal are still very much established in its culture and are considered essential forms of education. In this context, this magistrate believes that physical punishment should be discouraged through "a decisive and clear pedagogical approach" (Id, p.71). In fact, children's rights stem from their vulnerability and adults' obligations to protect them.

1.2.1 - Concept and Types

The concepts used by the scientific community and professionals in general to identify child/adolescent abuse do not always coincide with the legal nomenclature of the crimes perpetrated in this area, which are provided for in the various legal systems of different countries (Magalhães, 2010).

In scientific and social research or in clinical practice, the concepts of mistreatment or abuse are often used:

> "any form of physical and/or emotional treatment, non-accidental and inappropriate, resulting from dysfunctions and/or deficiencies in interpersonal relationships, in the context of a relationship of dependence (physical, emotional, psychological), trust and power. It can manifest itself through active behaviour (physical, emotional or sexual) or passive behaviour (omission or neglect of care or affection). Because of the repeated way in which they usually occur, they deprive the victim of their rights and freedoms, concretely or potentially affecting their health, dignity or development (physical, psychological and social). Such behaviour should be analysed in terms of
> the culture and time in which they take place" (Magalhães, 2005, p.32).

These abuses can be categorised according to the context in which they occur:

- intrafamilial violence, which is described in the literature as mistreatment and situations known as "domestic violence" (Magalhães, 2010, p.7);

- extra-familial when infringed in institutions or in the context of a care relationship (Magalhães, 2010, p.7).

Establishing clear boundaries between the various forms of child abuse is a difficult task, given that each one is not perfectly watertight. A situation of physical abuse can occur simultaneously with psychological abuse, but the reverse may not be true (Azevedo; Maia, 2006). Most children who are victims of these forms of aggression can be subjected to various types of abuse, which need to be examined separately, given the fact pointed out by English; Bangdwala; Runyan (2005) that the antecedent and consequent factors of each form of abuse manifest themselves differently.

Abuse can be the result of an omission or an action and can coexist in different types. For the purposes of this research, the following types are important: physical, sexual and emotional, neglect and Munchausen Syndrome by proxy (Dias, 2004; Ribeiro, 2009; Magalhães, 2010).

The WHO (2006) defines physical abuse as the intentional use of physical force against a child, which causes damage to their health, survival, development and dignity. It involves the assault or beating of a child, who may suffer various types of trauma such as bruising, haematomas, burns, fractures, suffocation, drowning, intoxication, traumatic brain injuries, internal organ damage and poisoning.

This includes shaken children, which can be carried out by parents or anyone else and has various manifestations. It is the most frequently diagnosed in health institutions, responsible for high morbidity and disability and the main cause of mortality (Magalhães, 2010).

Sexual abuse can take the form of involving a child in practices aimed at the sexual satisfaction of an adult or older young person who exercises a position of power or authority over them, usually under duress or threat. It includes various types of activities, from exhibitionism, photography, films

pornography, contact with the sexual organs, up to the consummation of the sexual act or other sexual practices (Magalhães, 2010).

The WHO (2006) considers this type of abuse to include cases in which the child is seen as an accomplice in situations of sexual violence perpetrated against them, sexual violence in intimate relationships, child marriage and harmful cultural practices such as genital mutilation (Ribeiro, 2009).

With regard to the definition of sexual abuse, it is important to consider that abusive situations may or may not have a coercive nature, whether or not physical and/or verbal threats are used (Browne; Finkelhor, 1986; Giarretto, 1982, cited by Carmo et al., 2002).

Negligence is defined as:

> "regular behaviour of omission, in relation to the necessary requests of the child or young person, not being provided with the satisfaction of their needs in relation to basic hygiene, food, safety, education, affection and health care, which results in damage to health and physical, emotional, moral or social development. It includes various forms: intrauterine, physical, psycho-affective or emotional, school, abandonment and begging" (Magalhães 2010, p.9).

Machado and Gonçalves (2002, p.21) consider that neglect arises when there is "an inability to provide the child with the basic needs of hygiene, food, affection, health and supervision", which are essential for the development, growth and well-being of the child/adolescent.

Azevedo and Maia (2006, p.33) state that neglect can happen consciously on the part of the aggressors, as well as through a "manifestation of ignorance, lack of information or training, poverty or parental inability to protect and care for children and young people".

Magalhães (2010) defines emotional abuse as an act of an intentional nature that is characterised by the persistent or significant, active or passive lack or omission of affective support and recognition of the emotional needs of the child/adolescent. This has the opposite effect on the development and stability of emotional and social competences, with a decrease in self-esteem. It can be manifested through verbal insults, humiliation, ridicule, devaluation, intimidation, hostility, rejection, lack of interest, discrimination, temporary abandonment, blaming, criticism and subjection to participation in situations of extreme or repeated domestic violence.

In the last two decades, this concept applied to children has been further developed. In addition to patterns of behaviour involving rejection, isolation, terrorism, disregard and/or corruption and deprivation of emotional response, deprivation of mental and physical health and educational neglect have been added (Myers et al., 2002). This form of violence is very common and the least identified, due to the high degree of social tolerance towards this type of abuse. Virtually nobody denounces or holds parents, relatives, teachers, police officers and health professionals, among others, responsible for disqualifying or humiliating children/adolescents (Magalhães, 2005).

It is worth pointing out that this type of abuse can be the only form of victimisation and can coexist with all the other situations of abuse mentioned above. Nevertheless, it should be invoked whenever it occurs (Magalhães, 2010).

With this in mind, psychological violence goes almost unnoticed, especially when the physical mark is visible.

Munchausen Syndrome by Proxy is "a situation in which a child is brought in for medical care, but the signs and symptoms they present are invented or provoked by their parents or carers" (Levy et al., 1986, p.31). They victimise the child by inflicting physical suffering, requesting unnecessary tests, using medication for no clinical reason and even causing psychological damage. It is a false disorder in which the action of simulating or producing a physical or psychological illness is directed at a third party, in most cases the child(ren), with the aim of obtaining attention from health professionals. It's a form of violence that is little known and also little diagnosed in Portugal. This syndrome affects not only the mother-child dyad, but the entire family spectrum, as there are real or simulated physical symptoms and the severity of the situation becomes greater (Ministério da Saúde, 2002).

The syndrome is difficult for professionals to diagnose, among other factors, because of the lack of knowledge about it, due to the scant literature on the subject (Feldman; Brown, 2007) and the aggressor's attitude of denying any kind of offence. In this sense, Forsyth (1995) believes that the more aware professionals are of the syndrome, the more cases will be diagnosed.

In order to better identify children and adolescents at risk, the bodies responsible for this, namely the National Commission for the Protection of Children and Young People at Risk (CNPCJR), have tried to conceptually operationalise other situations of danger such as: school drop-out and abandonment, exploitation of child labour and begging.

Abandonment is a type of mistreatment of which the child/adolescent is a victim from the very first day of their life. They can be abandoned in hospitals or maternity wards, locked up at home and left on the street, without their basic human needs and safety being ensured (CNPCJR, 2005). These include hunger, lack of protection from the cold, the need for hygiene and health care. Wounds and various and frequent illnesses are some of the signs and symptoms of children who have been abandoned. Dropping out of school occurs when a child/adolescent leaves compulsory basic education between the ages of six and fifteen (CNPCJR, 2005).

In Portugal, Decree-Law 176/2012 extended the age of compulsory education to 18 and enshrined the universality of pre-school education for children from the age of five.

Child labour exploitation includes any situation in which a child/adolescent is forced to do work that is beyond their limits, which should be done by adults, and which will interfere with their school activities and needs. In this case, indicators such as: the minor's participation in labour activities (on a regular or sporadic basis and the impediment to participating in school and social activities appropriate to their age) should be taken into account (CNPCJR, 2005).

It is important to remember that the majority of children/adolescents who work before the age allowed by law (Art. 66 of the Labour Code) are deprived of basic health care, education, nutrition, protection and security by their families (CNPCJR, 2005). Victims of exploitation are often simultaneously victims of ill-treatment and physical and psychological violence in the workplace.

Begging includes children who are used to beg on a regular or sporadic basis, or who do so of their own free will.

The complexity of the phenomenon of intra-family and extra-family violence against children/adolescents requires articulation and joint work between the different sectors of society in order to find more effective ways of preventing, detecting and dealing with these situations (Gonçalves, 2003).

1.2.2 - Epidemiology of abuse

Establishing the number of child/adolescent victims who are exposed to abuse within the family "is a complex and controversial endeavour due to a variety of conceptual and procedural reasons" (Berman et al., 2004 p.151). Much of the statistical data, particularly at the intra-family level, presented by institutions, are estimates calculated on the basis of detected situations (Catarino, 2007).

It is risky to assert the incidence of abuse, given the vulnerability of the child/adolescent, their dependence on the abuser and the fact that it occurs in a family context. In addition, there is the social legitimacy of its practice, especially if it is associated with educational practice and the difficulties of identifying and signalling abuse (Id, 2007).

With regard to identification/signalling, there is underreporting of intrafamily abuse against children/adolescents:

- there is a kind of social acceptance of violence used as a justification for "educating", especially when it does not produce visible and lasting physical damage (Ramos, 2011);
- fear of getting involved and of the aggressor's reactions (parents, relatives, carers);
- belief about what happens in the family environment is private, of interest only to those who are part of the environment and should not be made public;
- effect of the measures adopted, people don't believe the results of the notification.

This mentality urgently needs to be revised, especially when abuse is a form of violence that takes place within families. It needs to be denaturalised and denounced, treating it as a challenge to be overcome that is everyone's responsibility (Ramos, 2011).

Incongruities in the classification of child deaths and the lack of common definitions of abuse mean that there are no internationally comparable data in this area (Magalhães, 2010).

The Innocenti Report Card 5 (UNICEF, 2003, p.1) considers that there is a "growing conviction that child mortality as a result of maltreatment is under-represented in the available statistics". The same report states that all this statistical data should be treated with caution and advocates the need to adopt consistent research methods in all countries to improve the data collection process. These measures make it possible to inform and guide child/adolescent protection policies.

Every year in developed countries, child abuse causes 3,500 deaths of children under the age of 15, with the youngest group being the most vulnerable. Countries such as Spain, Greece, Italy, Ireland and Norway appear to have an exceptionally low incidence of child abuse deaths. In contrast, Belgium, the Czech Republic, New Zealand, Hungary and France have levels four to six times higher. The United States, Mexico and Portugal have rates 10 to 15 times higher than the first countries mentioned (Unicef, 2003).

The annual reports evaluating the activities carried out by the CPCJ show that the number of child and adolescent danger situations signalled in recent years in Portugal has been on the rise (CNPCJR, 2011, p.27). The majority of these situations are of five types: "neglect, exposure to deviant behaviour models, dangerous situations that jeopardise the right to education and psychological/emotional and physical abuse". With regard to the signalling bodies, in descending order, in 2011 the reports came from educational establishments, police authorities, parents/carers and the CPCJR (CNPCJR, 2011).

In the first half of 2013, the CPCJs monitored 53494 children/adolescents, of which they closed 13294 (24.85%). There was a difference of 541 fewer cases between the total number of active cases in 2012 (n=35628) and the number of cases that were carried over to 2013 (n=35087), which is less than that recorded in the previous year (n=1877).

Of the total number of children/adolescents characterised, 65.59% (n=35087) are children with cases in progress, 27.9% (n=14930) with cases opened, and 6.49% (n=3166) with cases reopened (Table 1).

Table 1- Evolution of the Procedural Flow in the CPCJ

	T	%	1	%	R	%	G	Arch	%	A	%
1° Without 2012	34832	50,47	14512	21,02	2822	4,08	52166	15054	21,81	37112	53,78
2° Without 2012	33605	48,69	14637	21,21	3431	4,97	No data	No data		No data	51,62
Year 2012	33605	48,69	29149	42,24	6253	9,06	69007	33379	48,37	35628	
1st Sem 2013	35087	65,59	14930	27,9	3477	6,49	53494	13294	24,85	40200	75,14

T=Transited; I=Initiated; R= Reopened; G= Global; Arq= Archived; A= Active Source: CNPCJR, 2013, p.2

In Portugal, in all age groups, the number of male children/adolescents (54.1 per cent) monitored by the CPCJ in the first half of 2013 was higher than the number of female children/adolescents (45.9 per cent) monitored in the same period (Table 2).

When analysing by age group, the 15 to 21 age group (18571) stands out as having the highest number of children/adolescents monitored, with 35.8% of the total. This age group has the highest figures for both sexes, with a 3.6 per cent difference between males and females, which means that 1,875 more children/adolescents are being looked after by males. It's worth mentioning that of the 1,871 young people monitored in this age group, 4,976 are aged between 18 and 21 (9.6% of the total).

It should be noted that this age group was the least representative in the report for the first half of 2012. However, in the 2012 Annual Report there had already been a reversal in the representation of age groups, with the 15/21 age group taking on a greater preponderance. This result is confirmed in the data for the first half of 2013 (CNPCJR, 2013).

The 11 to 14 age group (1,197) came in second place, accounting for 23.5 per cent of all children/adolescents monitored. In this age group, the difference between the two sexes is 2.9 per cent, which translates into 1,529 more male children and young people being monitored (Id, 2013).

In third place in the total number of children in care is the 6 to 10 age group, with 21.0 per cent (10897). In this age group, the percentage and absolute differences between the two sexes are smaller, with 1.3 per cent (6663) more male children and young people being accompanied (Id, 2013).

Lastly, the 0-5 age group represents 19.7 % (10,222) of the total number of children accompanied. It should be noted that in this age group, the number of children accompanied from 0 to 2 years old, 4,464, (males 2,274; females 2,090) accounted for 42.7 per cent, less than half of the total for this age group and 8.4 per cent of the total number of children and young people accompanied in the first half of 2013.

As we pointed out with regard to the 15/21 age group, we see a reversal in the statistical preponderance of the age groups when compared to the first half of 2012, but in line with what was seen in the 2012 Annual Report. It should be noted, however, that the 0-5 age group has moved up to 4th place, whereas in the 2012 annual report it was 3rd (CNPCJR, 2013).

Table 2 Distribution of children/adolescents monitored by the CPCJ according to gender and age group

AGE GROUP (YEARS)	1º SEMESTER 2012					1º SEMESTER 2013				
	F	%	M	%	Total	F	%	M	%	Total
0-5	8693	48,18	9348	51,82	18041	5038	49,28	5184	50,72	10222
6-10	7095	45,01	8665	54,99	15760	5117	46,95	5780	53,05	10897
11-14	8345	45,79	9876	54,11	18221	5334	43,73	6863	56,26	12197
15-21	5208	47,54	5746	52,46	10954	8348	44,95	10223	55,05	18571

Source: CNPCJR, 2013,p.6

This brief epidemiological analysis is an incentive to reflect on the scope of this problem and the nursing intervention to be carried out in favour of protecting and promoting the rights of children/adolescents.

1.2.3 - Risk Factors

Understanding the historical evolution, concept, typology and epidemiological context of child/adolescent abuse has allowed us to question the factors and mechanisms that contribute to its occurrence. Knowing these factors facilitates the identification of individuals in danger and the design of strategies aimed at reducing risks (Matos; Figueiredo, 2001) and acting downstream and upstream of abuse situations (Dias, 2004).

Factors are conditions, elements or indicators that favour situations of abuse, increasing their likelihood of occurrence when they occur simultaneously. The nature of these indicators is multiple and can be individual - parents/carers, child/adolescent, development/growth - and contextual - social, cultural, economic, family, specific life experiences or the environment - (Martinet, 2007).

The indicators for parents/carers include:

- addictions, such as alcoholism and drug addiction;
- physical and mental health disorders, with a history of deviant behaviour, personality changes - immaturity, impulsiveness, low self-control and self-esteem, low frustration tolerance and vulnerability to stress;

- incoherence in educational attitudes, a history of child abuse, very young age, especially maternal, very close pregnancies and disturbances in the attachment process;
- an excessive social or working life that makes it difficult to establish positive relationships with their children;
- the low social, economic and cultural level;
- unemployment and lack of knowledge about the child/adolescent development process (Magalhães, 2005).

The relationship between parents and/or carers and the child/adolescent can be influenced by the presence of one or more of the following indicators inherent to the child/adolescent themselves:

- vulnerability intrinsic to age and needs;
- personality and temperament not in tune with their parents;
- difficulties in managing emotions;
- prematurity and low birth weight;

- mental and physical health problems;
- under the age of three;
- sex;
- the result of an unwanted pregnancy;
- twin children;
- not living up to their parents' expectations;
- disabled or chronically ill children and children who have failed at school make them more vulnerable to victimisation (Magalhães, 2005);
- the influence of the peer group, race, religion and the media (Miller; Fox, *1987).*

Indicators of the family context include sources of family tension, unwanted pregnancy, family typology - single-parent, rebuilt with children from other relationships, large, or broken, with marital dysfunction or crisis situations - and families with serious socio-economic and housing problems (Magalhães, 2005). In relation to the family context, the studies carried out by:

w Weinraub and Wolf (1987 cited by Nunes 2009) state that the existence of a single carer, combined with the economic level, low social support and high levels of stress to which parents are subjected, can have negative consequences for the child/adolescent.

- Baer (1999, cited by Sousa, 2005) found significant differences in the levels of conflict between single-parent and nuclear families, noting that in the former, communication was perceived by the child as less satisfactory. He also added that the increased vulnerability of single-parent families leads to a deterioration in the parental role. In this context, children may not have basic security, so they internalise insecure attachment models, which hinder the process of autonomy and peaceful exploration of the environment. In these cases, they described the fragility of these children in terms of physical health and emotional well-being.

Abuse is particularly associated with both a climate of family violence and a dysfunctional relationship between parents and children. When children/adolescents experience a violent family member, they tend to adopt the same behaviour in their interpersonal relationships with peers (Peixoto, 2007).

- Sudbrack (1996) identified rigid standards of discipline, lack of negotiation with adolescents, addictive behaviour, lack of knowledge about adolescence, lack of guidance and control and pressure to work as risk indicators for adolescents.

Of the social and cultural context indicators, Magalhães (2005) pointed to social attitudes as a risk factor:

- the child being considered property, the value, rights and duties attributed, and socio-political concerns about childhood;
- the family, by emphasising the right to protection and privacy, considers the family environment to be the best choice for the child/adolescent to live in, and parental authority to be seen as a duty or a right;

- the violent behaviour, highlighting the penal framework and the characteristics of the victim support networks.

Magalhães (2005), based on Furniss (1991) and Briere (1992) for the importance they attach to assessing the severity of the abuse, considered the factors that intensify the trauma, such as (a):

- "early start;
- duration and frequency of abuse;
- degree of violence involved;
- occurrence of vaginal or anal penetration, in the case of sexual abuse;
- the occurrence of multiple abuses by different individuals;
- a marked difference between the ages of the abuser and the victim;
- degree of secrecy established between the abuser and the victim" (Id, p.47).

Several studies, including those by Atkinson and Hills (1998); Duncan and Brooks-Gunn, (1997); Luthar (1999); McLoyd (1998); Bynner (2001); Nelson et al. (2007), point to the following predictors of behavioural problems in children/adolescents, when they are carried out by parents, relatives or carers:

- behavioural disorders;
- oppositional defiant disorder;
- disruptive behaviour;
- externalisable problems.

These studies also point to the type of parenting and the development of social behaviours as reasonable/good predictors of the child's/adolescent's future.

The identification of risk factors is underpinned by intervention-orientated models. This is the case with the organisational model developed by Belsky (1980, cited by Magalhães, 2010), based on the concepts of Brofenbrenner (1974), which describes four ecological levels to consider in situations of child/adolescent abuse, emphasising a set of risk factors in each one:

- The microsystem refers to the family environment, as it is the most immediate context in which abuse occurs, emphasising the type of interactions developed between the child and the parents, marital conflicts, adaptability and cohesion of family relationships (Martinez Roig; Paul, 1993);
- mesosystem that includes the interrelationships between two or more elements in which the person and the family play an active role (Garbarino, 1992);
- exosystem in which the family does not interact directly, but includes, for example, social support networks and in which the stress caused by employment or unemployment stands out as risk factors (Azevedo; Maia, 2006);
- macrosystem influences the other systems. It is made up of the global pattern of ideology and organisation of social institutions common to a given culture or subculture (Bronfenbrenner, 1996).

This model has the virtue of situating child/adolescent abuse in the different contexts where it occurs, emphasising the level of intervention and the risk factors associated specifically with each one. In analysing and intervening in this phenomenon, Belsky (cited by Azevedo; Maia, 2006) considers individual variables, the formal and informal context of abusive families, and at the same time understands how the latter influences the other ecological levels.

1.3- NURSES' PRACTICES AND BEHAVIOURS

Promoting the rights and protection of children/adolescents at risk has posed new challenges for health services. According to the Directorate-General for Health (DGS, 2007, p.17) "risk situations refer to the potential danger to the realisation of the child's rights" in relation to their safety, health, training, education and development, so early detection of children at risk is undoubtedly the best way to prevent the potential danger that leads to situations of abuse.

The Regulation of Professional Nursing Practice (REPE) explains nursing as a profession that, in the area of health, aims to provide care to healthy or sick human beings throughout the life cycle and to the social groups in which they are integrated, at the levels of primary, secondary and tertiary prevention (DL no. 104/98, p.1754). The aim is for individual (child/adolescent) and group (family/community) clients to maintain, improve and recover their health and their maximum functional capacity.

Autonomous and interdependent nursing interventions within the three levels of prevention tend to encourage clients to adopt healthy lifestyles. In this context, nurses are faced with families who need help in acquiring parenting skills. This requires a philosophy of providing family-centred care, in order to "help mothers/fathers acquire the skills associated with an effective exercise of the parental role, which seems to us to build a proactive and constructivist dimension of health care delivery systems (Silva, 2011, p.920).

In order to help promote adequate child development, nurses must interact in accordance with the structure, functions, roles and expectations of the family and the behaviours and values of the society in which they live (Lima, 2009). At the same time as supporting "children with special needs, at risk or especially vulnerable, reducing inequalities in access to health services and recognising parents as primary caregivers are key aspects" (DGS, 2013, p.10).

Nurses specialising in child health nursing and paediatrics play an important role in helping clients adapt to changes in their health and family dynamics. To do this, they need to have the competences (knowledge and skills) to anticipate and respond to the needs of the child/adolescent, family and community (OE, 2010).

The professional performance of this specialist maximises the potential of human development, the management of well-being, early detection, the referral of dangerous situations, the promotion of self-esteem and health decision-making (OE, 2010).

This is reinforced by Almoarqueg et al. (1999), who emphasise the ability of these professionals to recognise situations of risk and/or evidence indicating a situation of abuse, participate in the data collection process, encourage the maintenance of an affective bond with the family, preserve ethics and protect against the manifestation of prejudice and violence, and guide family members in basic health care, based on the nursing focus of attention.

In the area of primary health care, nursing interventions take the form of the following activities/programmes aimed at individual clients and/or groups: home visits (HV), child health consultations and school health programmes (DGS, 2002).

Nurses are able to identify risk situations, refer abused children and promote children's health, through nursing HV for newborns (after hospital discharge), nursing consultations as part of child health surveillance, integrated into compliance with the child and adolescent health programme, from birth to adolescence, and encouragement to comply with the national vaccination plan, through to school health programmes, developed in partnership with educational establishments at various levels (OE, 2009).

The DGS, in 2002, valued nursing HV when it expanded human and material resources to make it a reality, as it considered it a basic element of health surveillance and promotion, particularly in the days following discharge from maternity hospital, in situations of prolonged or chronic illness and in cases of families or situations identified as being at risk.

DV provides insight into family dynamics, focussing on the relationships established between family members, economic and housing conditions, family resources and support, and identifying parental competences that put the child/adolescent at risk (Kulik et al., 2011).

The nursing consultation, up to 15 days of life, is one of the moments in nursing practice that provides information or indicators to get to know the family - for example, structures, functions - identify/evaluate individual, family and contextual risk factors and establish preventive measures aimed at the child/adolescent who is a victim or at risk of abuse. In addition, during the assessment, the nurse must combine the subjective and/or objective data observed and/or provided by the parents and/or carers in the clinical history report (Algeri, 2007; Kalik, 2011).

School health programmes make it possible to promote individual and collective health, which comes from "education, behaviour and lifestyles, chronic disease management and therapeutic alliance, as well as strengthening the power and responsibility of citizens to contribute to improving individual and collective health" (PNS, 20112016, p.3). The activities of these programmes should be based on interventions based on scientific evidence, aimed in particular at children and adolescents (Gaspar et al., 2009; Pinto et al., 2009; WHO, 2010) and on practices and strategies that make it possible to modify risk behaviours in order to promote the well-being and safety of children and young people.

Health Education (EPS) goes beyond the informative approach, as it involves the acquisition of healthy attitudes and behaviours. The practices and strategies used can favour the reversal of attitudes and experiences for the benefit of individual, family and community well-being and facilitate self-knowledge and knowledge of the environment (Mosquera; Stobaus, 1984).

The development of EPS combined with the promotion of assertive skills in clients can increase awareness and exert a positive influence on risk behaviours (Brito, 2009). Corroborating this idea, Ferreira (2008) and Ferreira (2011) add that primary health care nurses should focus on community health, given the favourable and unique position they are in to promote the health of children and adolescents, individually and/or as a group. Their vulnerability makes them ideal targets for prevention programmes (Breda, 2010; Simões, 2001, cit. by Fernandes, 2012).

The approach to child/adolescent victims of abuse and their families requires:

- "A programme of nursing action in child abuse should be part of child health surveillance, the purpose of which is to systematically collect the actions to be taken in cases of abuse and standardise them" (DIAZ HUERTAZ et al., 2001, cited by Catarino 2007, p.56);
- an attitude of genuine empathy, respect and kindness because, most of the time, the intervention is aimed at reorganising family ties (Brasil, 2002; SBP/FIOCRUZ/MJ, 2001).

Gary and Humphreys (2004) consider that these characteristics of nurses are essential for establishing a therapeutic relationship with their clients, as it is their primary role to educate the population at every possible opportunity and contact, thus contributing to the prevention of the phenomenon of intrafamily violence (Mosquera; Strobaus, 1984).

In the area of child abuse, the EPS programmes cover five areas of action:

- Training, in which the courses were aimed at acquiring knowledge about childhood, risk and abuse indicators and the techniques of the comprehensive intervention approach in childhood/adolescence;
- The recording of cases of risk and child abuse. To this end, an identification sheet has been created with the indicators of child abuse, enabling them to be recorded quickly and reliably;
- Diagnosis and specialised intervention to identify suspected cases and assess the extent of the injuries to the abused child/adolescent and the recovery of the family unit when possible;
- Prevention, based especially on more favourable moments in life such as pregnancy, birth and the first years of life, which require greater monitoring of the child's/adolescent's development and growth.
- The development of guidelines (Catarino, 2007; DGS, 2013).

In situations of child abuse, HV, nursing consultations and school health programmes play a key role, as they are ideal moments for developing clients' skills and healthy behaviours/attitudes, depending on their reality.

In situations of abuse, the nature of the facilitating or inhibiting factors is diverse and interrelated, and can be systematised into three dimensions: individual, professional and the problem inherent in the abuse.

The difficulty in identifying and managing situations of abuse, as an individual condition, is associated with feelings of uncertainty, anger, projection, anxiety and impotence, which seem to be related to the professional's defence mechanisms to minimise their suffering (Silva, 2011).

In this sense, nurses have to

> "having interpersonal skills - a stabilised professional and personal life; the ability to accept others without prejudice; sociability; an active interest in people and in finding new solutions; the ability to take an interest in family problems without getting personally involved - and cultural mastery -

knowledge of how cultural factors influence the appearance of abuse; understanding the concept of the family in each culture and the different life choices based on cultural factors" (Magalhães, 2005, p.105).

This same difficulty can arise in relation to the professional constraints that come with it:

- the position of professionals, often interposed by fear and ignorance of the magnitude of the situation and/or the social impact on the life of the child/adolescent and their family;
- This is due to the need for nurses to acquire a theoretical and analytical framework that allows them to understand the problem, its complexity and the different ways in which it manifests itself. This training can be obtained through continuous in-service education (Silva et al., 2011). Magalhães (2005, p.105) suggests the existence of specific training in order to provide them with technical skills and experience (inclusion of this subject in the course curriculum; training courses and actions; internships);
- of interdisciplinary teamwork involving health professionals, education and legal authorities and requires a transversal approach to knowledge, policies and social practices in the technical operationalisation of interventions based on programmes and projects that go beyond institutions (Magalhães, 2005; Marsland, 1994, cited by Scherer, 2000; DGS, 2011);
- the human and material resources available (Magalhães, 2005);
- how to assess the validity and reliability of programmes.

And finally, this difficulty can be related to conditions inherent to the problem of abuse, particularly of a technical and ethical nature:

- the complexity of child abuse explanatory models;
- the relative lack of knowledge of the "real" factors at work in each situation and the limited ability to predict and detect the supposed risk factors (Silva, 2011);
- the fact that many potential aggressors don't actually carry out the abuse;
- the danger of violating the privacy of the child/adolescent and/or family (Canha, 2003; Alberto, 2006; Azevedo; Maia, 2006).

The complexity of abuse situations has led professionals to construct a guiding principle that facilitates the development of the child's/adolescent's capacities and potential (DGS, 2013) and to record the notification. Reporting is mandatory because of the damage caused to the victim's health, the criminal aspect of abuse and, above all, because it is an instrument for protecting and defending victimised children and adolescents (Maranhão, 2005; Silva, 2006; Cunha, 2007).

This complexity, which is intrinsic to situations of abuse and the current level of knowledge about them, conditions the intervention of health professionals before they occur. Therefore, developing an effective preventive strategy based on the aetiology of abuse situations is a difficult but priority task (Paul; Arrubarrena, 1996; Magalhães, 2010). This strategy can be described in three levels of prevention: primary, secondary and tertiary (Caplan, 1964; Magalhães, 2005; Alberto, 2006; Azevedo; Maia, 2006).

Prevention, in general, encompasses a set of strategies that aim to prevent the appearance of unhealthy and maladjusted behaviours, protect and support individuals who are on the verge of taking on risky behaviours and, finally, recover and reintegrate those who are already in danger or have been victims, i.e. those who exhibit problem behaviours (Matos et al., 1997). In this sense, prevention is a noble and difficult nursing activity, but it should always be at the forefront of professional performance (Leandro, 1999).

Primary prevention targets the general population and acts before any manifestation of abuse, taking into account social, economic and family situations, among others. To this end, it is necessary to develop actions in the areas of research, professional training and public awareness/information; changes and adjustments to the legal framework and the creation of specific services (Canha, 2000). These actions are aimed at:

r reducing situations that favour the emergence of addictive behaviours, eliminating poverty, reducing unwanted pregnancies and reducing situations of social isolation (Id, 2000).

• changing existing attitudes in society towards the use of corporal punishment, reducing violent family relationships and increasing knowledge about the real needs, both physical and psychological, of children/adolescents.

Prevention implies acting for the whole, considering the different systems of human development (Brofenbrenner, 2002) regardless of the existence or not of risk factors (Azevedo and Maia, 2006; Alberto, 2006), that is:

> "to emphasise community and be interdisciplinary, to be proactive and interconnect the different aspects of people's lives with a biopsychosocial orientation, to use education and social techniques more than individual ones, to aim to provide people with the environmental and personal resources to face problems on their own and to promote the existence of fair social contexts" (Casa 1994, cited by Paul; Arruabarrena, 1996, p.330).

This approach is ambitious and generalised, and the results can only be assessed in the long term. However, its application would lead to a reduction in the risk that produces situations of lack of protection and an improvement in the quality of life in childhood and adolescence (Paul; Arruabarrena, 1996).

Programmes that integrate primary prevention must give children/adolescents the tools to recognise and avoid dangerous situations. It is essential that nurses:

• establish a close relationship with the child/adolescent in the places they go to, for example, school institutions and sports associations;

• build spaces for family members to reflect on the problem, providing information on the characteristics of a dangerous situation, the consequences and the recommended intervention (Canha, 2003; Alberto, 2006);

• guide the family in the development of the child/adolescent in a way that favours the bond between them (Gonçalves, 2003).

Nurses, members of the multidisciplinary team, are essential in identifying situations of risk and/or victims of abuse, due to their privileged position in the relationship with the community and their autonomy in making decisions to resolve these situations (Algeri, 2007).

Secondary prevention aims to identify and provide services to social groups at risk, in order to prevent the emergence of psychosocial, family and/or individual factors that lead to the problem (Caplan, 1964; Paul and Arruabarrena, 1996; Magalhães, 2005; Alberto, 2006; Azevedo and Maia, 2006). This preventive practice requires nurses to be able to predict the aggressive behaviour of a subject or family with a high probability of being an aggressor towards a child/adolescent (Azevedo; Maia, 2006).

As part of secondary prevention, nurses can develop autonomous and interdependent interventions to empower parents - knowledge and skills - to cope better with the demands of parenthood and manage the stress associated with performing the parental role; strengthen attachment bonds; guide parents of children with special educational needs and refer all family members to social and health services (Paul; Arruabarrena, 1996).

It is desirable that any investment in society's health gains be focussed on implementing preventive strategies at primary and secondary level, in order to result in fewer situations of abuse. However, the current reality does not fit into this framework, since a large part of these efforts are centred on tertiary prevention. The aim of tertiary prevention is to reduce the duration of the abuse and the severity of the consequences, to rehabilitate and integrate the child/adolescent (victim) and their family into the community (Canha, 2003; Alberto, 2006; Azevedo; Maia, 2006).

In this context, the use of the term prevention becomes questionable, because the interventions developed at this level come after the situation of abuse has occurred. However, by preventing the recurrence and/or reproduction of abuse situations, nurses implicitly prevent a set of consequences arising from these situations (Paul; Arruabarrena, 1996).

Nursing interventions in tertiary prevention must guarantee the safety and physical and psychological integrity of the child/adolescent victim of abuse, in order to avoid re-victimisation or chronic abuse (Canha, 2003; Alberto, 2006; Azevedo; Maia, 2006). It is also important to consider high-risk individuals with a history of previous abuse as potential aggressors, since their vulnerable condition as a victim can turn into a form of abuse as an aggressor (Paul; Arruabarrena, 1996).

These three levels of prevention must be developed from an integrated perspective in order to combat abuse. The strategies to be implemented must be based on the reality of each child/adolescent, family and community, in order to promote the cultural, normative and economic changes needed to avoid dysfunctional environments that can lead to abuse (Reis, 2009).

In short, nurses' practice in situations of abuse must be guided by breaking the silence and professional accommodation and by understanding the contradictions of the power relations that make up a hierarchical and unequal social order, in which relations of gender, class, race, age, among others, are mixed (Catarino, 2007).

We highlight the responsibility of the Paediatric and Child Health Specialist Nurse to ensure the well-being of the child/adolescent, as part of a family and community, by "providing nursing care that requires a deeper level of knowledge and skills, acting specifically with the user (individual, family or group) in situations of crisis or risk, within the scope of their speciality" (DL n°437/91, p.5725).

CHAPTER 2

METHODOLOGICAL FRAMEWORK

One of the most important phases of any research work is the methodological definition, as it includes all the elements that help give the research a path or direction (Freixo, 2011).

Society has evolved thanks to the progress of research in different areas of knowledge, to which nursing as a science and profession has not been oblivious. Nursing research makes it possible to obtain answers to the questions posed by professionals in their daily practice, in order to discover new knowledge that is essential to the quality of care, the updating of techniques and protocols implemented and the improvement of nurses' skills (Fortin, 2009).This chapter presents the empirical part of the work, where we present the methodology used, describe the procedures carried out and the justifications for the choices made.

2.1 - JUSTIFICATION AND PURPOSE OF THE STUDY

The changes that have taken place in societies have contributed to an improvement in the resolution of the problem of child and adolescent abuse, despite the fact that violence has always been part of the human experience and that sometimes the demands for an immediate return on public investment make it impossible to implement programmes to prevent this type of situation.

It is essential to systematically implement tools that allow for gains in prevention, early detection and diagnosis, and in decision-making at the level of an interdisciplinary intervention plan for each child, from a holistic perspective, valuing all their psychological, biological, social, cultural and spiritual dimensions, while also taking into account the family and the surrounding social environment (Penha, 1996). However, we realise that diagnosing and intervening in situations of child/adolescent abuse is not always easy. The frequency and seriousness of the cases that arise on a daily basis prove this. Recognising that detection
These situations are a social, ethical and legal requirement and the whole process of child protection is assumed to be a fundamental priority (Azevedo; Maia, 2006). As a nurse in the area of child and adolescent health and a member of the NACJR, we have an added responsibility to promote positive changes in the community where we work, in terms of health education on children at risk and child abuse and in improving intervention.

The CSP is one of the most important places for effective measures to prevent and control risk factors and to enhance protective factors against child abuse (Catarino, 2007). The activities carried out provide opportunities to observe signs of child abuse or neglect, and nurses are in a privileged position to detect these situations. Therefore, they should not resign themselves to being promoters of child welfare and taking an active role in the prevention and diagnosis of abuse. It is important to consider that there may be factors that interfere with their ability to identify and signal child abuse, such as fear on the part of professionals and lack of knowledge of the real magnitude (Magalhães, 2010).

The decision to study nurses' practices, behaviours and knowledge of child and adolescent abuse is related to my work as a nurse at the NACJR, the concern shown by colleagues in dealing with this problem and the interest in cooperating to improve the nursing care provided to children/adolescents.

The study aims to contribute to excellence in nursing care for children and adolescents, with a view to minimising the perpetuation of abuse.

2.2 - Research question

The first challenge for the researcher is to be able to express what is a focus of interest or a difficulty that they are facing and that they want to resolve through relevant, feasible and explicit research. Clarifying the problem by formulating the starting question allows the researcher to "express as precisely as possible what they are trying to know, elucidate and understand better" (Quivy; Campenhoudt, 2008, p.32).

The research questions defined were as follows:

- What are the practices and behaviours of PHC nurses when dealing with abused children and adolescents?
- What knowledge do nurses have about child and adolescent abuse?
- What are nurses' training needs on child abuse?

2.3 - Objectives

The objective is "the main intention of a project, i.e. it corresponds to the end product that the project wants to achieve" (Sousa and Baptista, 2011, p.25-26).

The objectives that guide this work are:

- To identify nurses' practices with child and adolescent victims of abuse;
- To identify nurses' behaviour towards child and adolescent victims of abuse;
- To identify nurses' knowledge of child abuse;
- Identify nurses' training needs on child abuse.

2.4 - Type of Study

The study was based on the quantitative paradigm and was exploratory, descriptive, correlational and cross-sectional.

An exploratory study "seeks to learn more about the phenomena under study (...) by trying to ascertain the characteristics of knowledge or situations. A given reality is explored however little is known about it" (Oliveira, 2002, p.15).

Descriptive research aims to "discover new knowledge, describe existing phenomena, determine the frequency of occurrence of a phenomenon in a given population or categorise information" (Fortin, 2009, p.34). It is based on the constant collection of data from a representative sample of a given population and aims to "provide an explanation of the problem in as much detail as possible" (Oliveira, 2009).

According to Fortin (2009, p.244) "the descriptive-correlational study aims to explore relationships between variables and describe them". In this study, the researcher is often in the presence of variables of which he is unaware of which may be associated with each other. "The establishment of relationships between variables allows the phenomenon studied to be circumscribed" (Id, 2009, p.244).

The study's approach in terms of time is cross-sectional, as the data was collected at a single point in time and its aim was to assess the frequency of an event and its risk factors in a given population (Fortin, 2009; Oliveira, 2009). The choice of a cross-sectional study was due to the time allotted for it to be carried out.

2.5 - Population

The target population is the set of elements that the researcher wishes to study and make generalisations about, with the accessible population being the cases that are available to take part in the study and that meet the inclusion criteria (Fortin, 2009).

The target population for this research was nurses working in PHC in Portugal. Since it was impossible to study the entire population, we considered nurses from the PHC of the Grande Porto VII-Gaia Health Centre Group as the accessible population.

There was no need to identify a sample, given that the accessible population was small (91 nurses) and could be studied in its entirety. Sampling is understood as "the procedure by which a group of people or a subset of a population is chosen in such a way that the entire population is represented" (Fortin, 2009, p.213).

We defined the inclusion criteria for the study as nurses providing care to children and adolescents in PHC.

The population was made up of nurses who agreed to take part in the research, totalling 91 participants.

2.6- Data Collection Instrument and Procedure

In a quantitative study, the questionnaire is one of the most widely used data collection methods, as it allows a large number of informants to be covered (Fortin, 2009), anonymity to be maintained and it is also a quick and economical way of obtaining information.

In this study we used Catarino's (2007) questionnaire "Child Maltreatment Practices and Behaviours of Nurses" (ANNEX III).

The instrument is made up of open, closed and mixed questions, and consists of three parts:

- The first includes the questions needed to characterise the nurses' socio-demographic and professional backgrounds (Questions 1 to 10), operationalised as follows:
  - **Age -** open question.
  - **Gender -** closed question, two categories: male and female.

- **Marital status -** closed question categorised into: single, married/marital partnership, separated/divorced and widowed.
- **Children** - dichotomous question: yes or no. Respondents who answered yes were asked to mention the number of children and their ages.
- **Academic qualifications - a** mixed question with the following answer options: Bachelor's degree or legal equivalent, Bachelor's degree or legal equivalent, Master's degree and PhD. For the last two options, the name of the qualification was requested.
- **Training -** closed question with two answer options: postgraduate, specialised.
- **Professional category** - closed question with four answer options: nurse, graduate nurse, specialist nurse and head nurse.
- **Place where you work** - closed question with eight answer options: Personalised Health Care Unit - headquarters, Personalised Health Care Unit - extension, Family Health Unit, Public Health Unit, Community Care Unit, Pneumological Diagnostic Centre, Canidelo Medical Centre and other.
- **Time in Professional Practice** - broken down into two open-ended questions to identify the length of time in professional practice and the length of time in CSP.
- The second part of the data collection instrument includes a scale made up of 25 items aimed at collecting data related to nurses' practices and behaviours in detecting and preventing child abuse and promoting child well-being and safety. It also includes questions designed to gather the information needed to understand the situations of danger identified by the participants who said they had already had contact with child victims of abuse.

The "Nurses' practices and behaviours in child abuse" scale takes the form of statements and asks participants to respond to the frequency of their practices and behaviours in detecting and preventing child abuse and promoting the child's well-being and safety. It is a five-point Likert scale, with 1 corresponding to Never, 2 to A few times, 3 to Sometimes, 4 to Often and 5 to Always. All the items were constructed in a positive sense, so the higher the score, the more often nurses carry out the correct practices and behaviours in the face of child abuse. The scale is made up of four sub-scales:

- Promoting child well-being and safety (PBESI) - 9 items (2,3,4,5,6,12,13,14,21);
- Tertiary prevention (PT) - 7 items (7,8,9,10,11,15,16);
- Early intervention for children and families at risk (IPCFR) - 4 items (1,17,18,19);
- Detecting and signalling child abuse (DSCMtI) - 5 items (20,22,23,24,25).

- **Contact with child victims of abuse -** closed-ended question operationalised as yes; no; I don't know. The aim is to collect data to assess whether the respondent has had contact with child victims of abuse during their professional activity.
- **Dangerous situations identified and action taken in response to the situation** identified - in order to ascertain the dangerous situations identified by the respondents who said they had been in contact with abused children, a multiple answer question was included with sixteen

response options: abandonment, neglect, school dropout, school absenteeism, physical abuse, psychological abuse, sexual abuse (suspected), abuse of authority, child labour, committing a criminal act, addictive behaviour, exposure to deviant behaviour models, begging, recurrent health problems, parental dysfunction, other, asking that if their option was this one, they identify which situation.

In order to understand the type of action taken by the nurse, they were asked to indicate the interventions they carried out for each situation of danger identified, among the 13 options suggested: involve the child to assess the situation, assess/monitor the child's behaviour, assess/monitor the child's physical condition, collect evidence for medico-legal assessment, teach the family safety measures, teach the importance of affective relationships, carry out a home visit to monitor the child and family, talk to the parents to confront and complete the information, refer to the family doctor, refer to social service technicians, report the situation, I didn't act, other, asking them to identify what type of intervention they had carried out.

- **Document used in the complaint -** mixed question with three categories: signposting guide, descriptive report and other, asking respondents whose answer choice was other to identify the type of document used.
- **Entity to which the complaint/contact was made -** mixed multiple-answer question with the following indicators: Security forces (PSP/GNR), other family member, psychologist, social service technician, NACJR, CPCJ, family doctor, emergency service, family and children's court, other, asking respondents in this last option to mention to which entity they made the complaint.
- **Existence of an identification document for families at risk -** closed question operationalised as: questionnaire, list of risks, don't know, other, asking respondents whose answer option was other to mention the type of document used.
- **Existence of a manual of procedures for situations of child abuse in the workplace** - closed question operationalised as yes, no and don't know.
- **Carrying out home visits to families at risk - a** dichotomous yes/no question aimed at finding out whether nurses carry out home visits to families at risk.
- **Contribution of home visits -** only for nurses who

responded to a home visit to find out their opinion, a multiple-answer question was posed asking them to indicate how it contributed. There were 15 answer options: increase the use of prenatal surveillance, improve the pregnant woman's nutritional status, reduce smoking during pregnancy and with the child, reduce the parents' drug and alcohol abuse, reduce the number of pregnancies and the spacing between them, reduce preterm labour, improve the newborn's birth weight, increase family attachment, improving the child's growth and development, reducing the criminal behaviour of carers, increasing the use of health and social services in the community, reducing the use of social aid, reducing the use of emergency services, reducing accidents and poisoning in children and carrying out EPS for children (each respondent could indicate more than one option).

- **Health education intervention related to child abuse -** question operationalised as yes or no, with the aim of finding out whether nurses carry out health education related to the topic of child abuse.

- **Themes addressed in the context of child abuse - an** open-ended question aimed at collecting data to identify the themes addressed by nurses in the context of abuse (only participants who mentioned carrying out health education answered this question).
- **Context of health education interventions** - mixed question with the aim of identifying the context in which health education interventions are developed, with the following indicators: nursing consultation, school health and HV.

- The third part of the data collection instrument covers questions aimed at gathering the information needed to identify nurses' training needs (Questions 1 to 5), with Questions 3 and 4 being single-item scales.

- **Specific training in the area of child abuse** - dichotomous question, yes/no, with the aim of finding out if the nurses have had specific training in the area of child abuse.
- **Training Context** - aimed at respondents who answered yes to the previous question, operationalised into: academic training, in-service training and self-training.
- **Self-perceived knowledge of child abuse** - closed-ended question. Respondents were asked, on a Likert scale from 1 to 5, to place an X on the option that best corresponded to their level of knowledge of child abuse, where 1 corresponded to No knowledge and 5 to A lot of knowledge.
- **Interest in obtaining further training in the area of child abuse** - closed question asking respondents to place an X on the option that best equated to their interest in the subject of child abuse, on a scale of 1 to 5. With 1 being No interest and 5 being Very interested.
- **Thematic areas of training** - multiple answer question, which aimed to identify the content that nurses consider most important to cover in training, categorised into seven options: communication techniques, diagnosis of child abuse, legal framework for child protection, family intervention programmes, school intervention programmes, community intervention programmes for at-risk groups, other (indicate which). Each participant could indicate more than one option.

The data was collected between February and March 2013, after authorisation from the executive director of the ACES (Appendix II).

Initially, the interlocutors from the different functional units were contacted and the objectives of the study were presented in person. Anonymity and data reliability were guaranteed. The material provided was read together: informed consent (appendix IV) and the questionnaire (appendix III), and any doubts were clarified and the researcher's contact details made available. The importance of completing the informed consent document in the research was emphasised. The questionnaire and the document for obtaining the participants' informed consent were distributed in envelopes by the nursing interlocutors of the different functional units of the ACES Grande Porto VII-Gaia (Personalised Health Care Unit - headquarters and extension, Family Health Unit, Public Health Unit, Community Care Unit, Pneumological Diagnostic Centre and Canidelo Medical Centre).

2.7- Data processing

Statistics is the science of collecting, analysing and interpreting data that varies (Beaglehole et al.1993; Triola, 2008). This science is involved in various stages of quantitative research. It is the type of research carried out, the type of variables and the research questions formulated that will determine the choice of statistical tool (Fortin, 2009).

The data was statistically analysed using SPSS (Statistical Package for Social Sciences) version 20 for Windows. According to Pereira (2008), this computerised tool is very useful in that it allows various statistical calculations to be made and results to be obtained very quickly.

The data collected was analysed using descriptive statistics, namely frequencies (absolute and relative), measures of central tendency (mean, mode and median) and measures of dispersion (standard deviation) and, at a later stage, inferential statistics.

Descriptive statistics make it possible to "describe the characteristics of the sample, how the data was collected and describe the values obtained by measuring the variables" (Fortin 1999, p.2779).

The measures of central tendency are a set of measures that help to describe the centre of the distribution of the values of a variable in the sample in question. The three most commonly used measures are the mode, mean and median. Measures of dispersion, on the other hand, are complementary measures for describing data that provide information on how close the individual values of the same variable are, or, on the contrary, how far they are from the centre of their distribution (Martins, 2011).

Inferential statistics allows us to "highlight the characteristics of a population based on data from a sample" (Fortin, 2009, p.440). In the inferential analysis, Student's t-test was used to assess nurses' practices and behaviours in relation to child abuse and academic qualifications and Pearson's correlation between the four sub-scales of the EPCEMtI and cronbach's alpha with $p < 0.05$.

2.8- Ethical and Legal Aspects

In a research process, ethics refers to the quality of the research techniques, with regard to the fulfilment of professional, legal or social obligations towards the subjects under study (Nunes, 2005).

Any research carried out with individuals raises ethical and legal issues, and the five fundamental principles or rights determined by the code of ethics must be taken into account, namely: the right to self-determination, intimacy, anonymity and confidentiality, protection from discomfort and harm, and fair and just treatment (Fortin, 2009).

These ethical principles were a constant concern for us, respecting the rights of the participants involved throughout this research. We therefore initially sought authorisation from the Executive Director of ACES Grande Porto VII-Gaia to carry out the research, explaining the information about the study. We received a favourable opinion (Appendix II). Data collection only began after approval.

Informed consent is essential in any research and is defined as the process by which researchers ensure that participants: receive full information about the study, make a free and informed decision whether or not to take part in it, are informed that they will not be harmed by accepting or refusing to take part and are informed of their right to anonymity and confidentiality (Nunes, 2005). Only nurses who signed this document (Appendix IV) took part in this study.

As previously mentioned, the questionnaire "Child Abuse, Practices and Behaviour of Nurses" by Catarino (2007) was used to carry out the research, after the author had duly requested permission and given her consent (ANNEX I).

After completing this journey, we committed ourselves to publicising the results to the institution involved in the research, as well as to the nurses in the different functional units.

CHAPTER 3

PRESENTATION, ANALYSIS AND DISCUSSION OF RESULTS

Once the information has been collected and organised, the results must be analysed and discussed in order to respond to the study's objectives. The first step in discussing the results is to characterise the population and present the research results, examining them in relation to the objectives and research questions. To present the data, tables, graphs and figures were used to illustrate the results.

3 1- Socio-demographic and Professional Characterisation

The study sample was made up of nurses from the different functional units of the ACES Grande Porto VII-Gaia, totalling 91 participants. They ranged in age from 22 to 65 (graph 1), with a mean (M) age of 36.92 years and a standard deviation (SD) of 9.12 years.

GRAPH 1 - Nurses' age

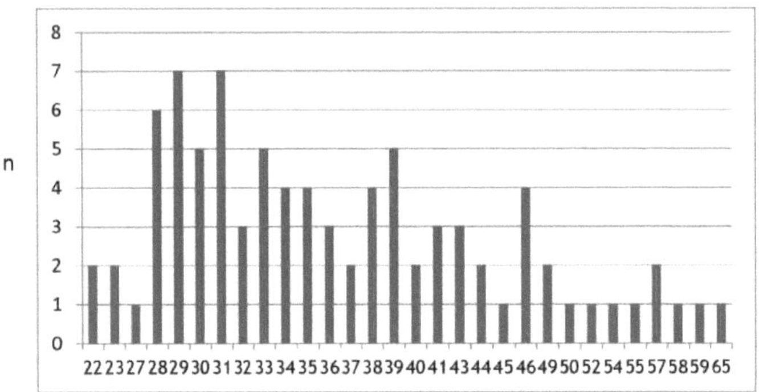

The majority (85.05%; n=78) are female, which confirms the historical trend of the profession, since it was women who ensured care, through knowledge passed down from generation to generation, since the dawn of humanity (Collière, 1989). This is also in line with the statistics from the OE (2012), which state that of the 65,467 nurses, 81.41% (n=53,301) are female.The participants are mostly married or living in a de facto union (60.47%; n= 55).

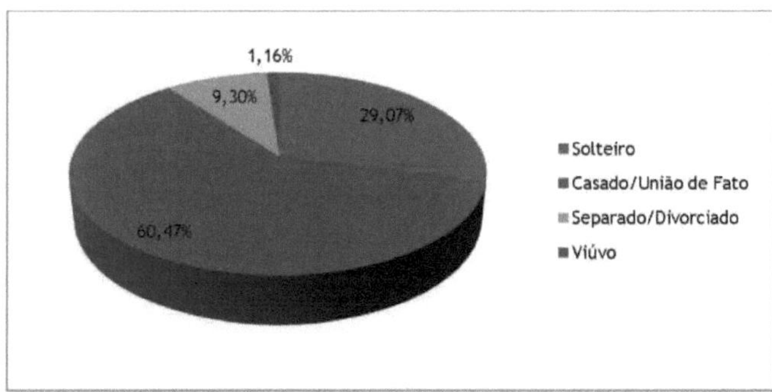

CHART 2 - Marital status

Of those surveyed, 63.5 per cent (n=58) have children, with the number varying between one and three and the age of the children between one year and thirty-six years (M=3 years and SD=0.72).

With regard to academic qualifications (graph 3), it was found that of the total number of respondents, the majority 77.01% (n=70) hold a degree in nursing or legal equivalent, 17.24% (n=16) hold a master's degree and 5.747% (n=5) hold a bachelor's degree or legal equivalent. These figures are in line with those presented by the OE (2012), which states that 81.15 per cent (n=53,131) of nurses hold only a bachelor's degree.

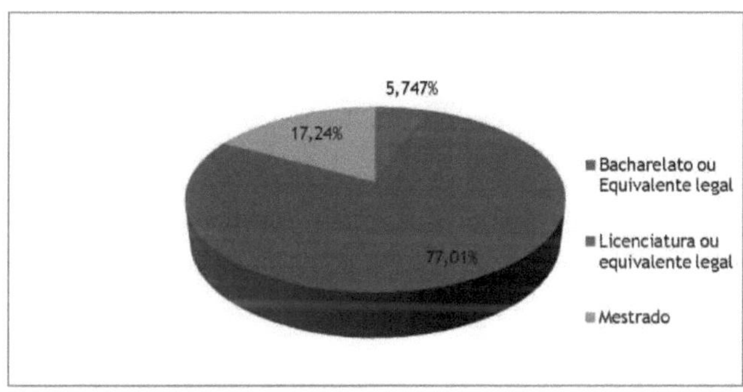

GRAPH 3- Academic qualifications

With regard to professional training (graph 4), 54.02% (n=49) of the respondents said they did not have any, 29.89% (n=27) had specialised training and 16.09% (n=15) had postgraduate training. The percentage of nurses with specialised or postgraduate training is higher than in the study by Catarino (2007), in which only 10.01% (n=6) nurses had training at this level.

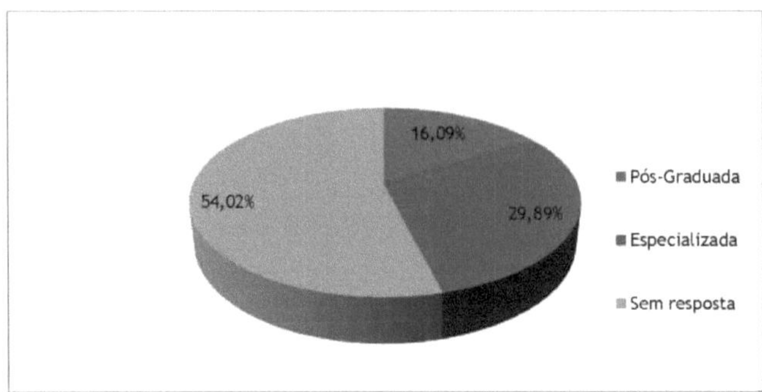

GRAPH 4- Professional training

With regard to professional category (graph 5), 44.83% (n=41) are nurses, 43.68% (n=40) graduate nurses and 11.49% (n=10) specialist nurses. These results are in line with the statistics from the OE (2012), which state that 18.86% (n=12,351) of nursing professionals are specialised nurses.

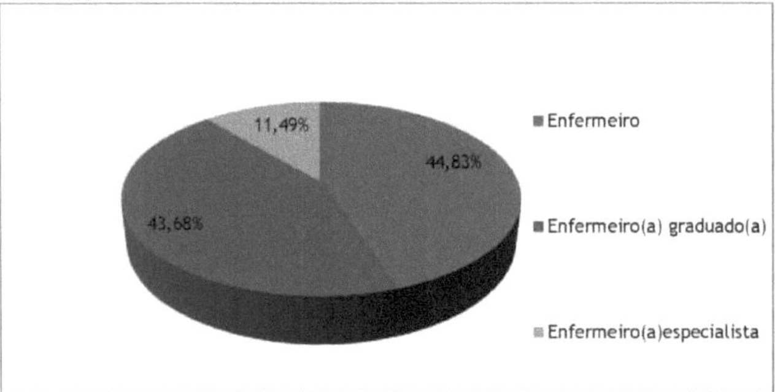

GRAPH 5 - Professional category

With regard to where they work (graph 6), the majority (55.29%; n=50) of the nurses surveyed work in family health units. The remaining 23.53% (n=21) work in the Personalised Health Care Units (UCSP) - headquarters - and a minority in the Pneumological Diagnostic Centre (CDP) and Public Health Unit (USP) - 1.176% (n=1.07). These figures differ from those of Catarino (2007), who found that the minority of nurses worked in USFs.

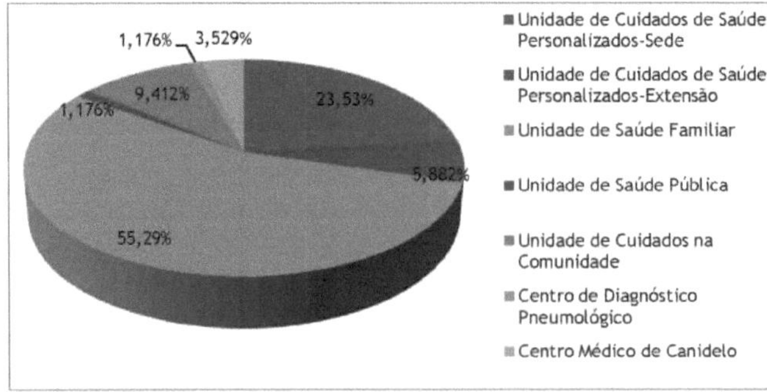

GRAPH 6 - Place of professional practice

The participants' length of professional practice (table 3) varied between one and 40 years (M=13.85; SD=8.701) and their length of practice in PHC varied between one and 35 years (M=8.63 years; SD=6.607).

TABLE 3 - Length of professional career

	N	Xmin	Xmax	M	Fashion	DP
Time in Professional Practice	91	1	40	13,85	10,00	8,701
Time worked in CSP	91	1	35	8,63	0,50	6,607

3.2- Nurses' Practices and Behaviours

With regard to the sensitivity of the EPCMtI, we can see in table 4 that the values obtained in our study are very similar to those of Catarino (2007).

Table 4 - EPCEMtl descriptive statistics

			Our Study				Catarino, 2007			
	Item		M	Md	Mo	DP	M	Md	Mo	DP
FATOR 1	2	I evaluate the quality of the mother/father/child emotional bond	1,93	2,00	2	0,90	2,21	2,00	2	0,934
	3	I assess the child's care and the presence of symptoms suggestive of abandonment or lack of affection	2,14	2,00	2	0,95	2,18	2,00	2	0,941
	4	I assess the attitude of parents towards setting educational standards and limits for their children	2,34	2,00	2	0,86	2,33	2,00	2	0,871
	5	I intervene with kindness and empathy, discussing alternative methods of discipline	2,23	2,00	2	0,85	2,34	2,00	2	0,835
	6	I promote the adequacy of the parental role and the self-esteem of parents	2,11	2,00	2	0,88	2,29	2,00	2	0,844
	12	I value the child's care in different health institutions (emergency, and/or permanent care)	2,44	2,00	2	1,05	2,42	2,00	2	0,973
	13	I value attitudes of detachment, detachment, deprivation of affection and security	1,97	2,00	2	0,86	2,02	2,00	2	0,770
	14	When observing the child, I look for the after-effects of the abuse (e.g. anxiety, social isolation, learning problems, behavioural changes).	2,51	2,00	2	0,99	2,41	2,00	2	0,864
	21	I observe the child's conduct and the parents' behaviour at appointments	1,75	2,00	1	0,85	**1,96**	2,00	1	0,920
	Total F1- Promoting child well-being and safety		**2,15**				**2,24**			
FATOR 2	7	I intervene in families at risk at an early, stable and continuous stage	2,96	3,00	3	1,06	2,95	3,00	3	0,910
	8	I work as part of a multidisciplinary team to continually assess the progress of the child and family.	2,47	2,00	2	1,06	2,71	3,00	2	0,992
	9	I recognise the mismatch between the child's history and injuries as physical abuse	2,56	3,00	3	0,97	2,41	2,00	2	0,844
	10	I value the delay in seeking health care for the child	1,92	2,00	2	0,84	2,15	2,00	2	0,898
	11	I value the injuries that the child presents at the different stages of development	2,05	2,00	2	1,01	2,12	2,00	2	0,940
	15	I identify the risk factors associated with child abuse	2,61	3,00	3	0,89	2,42	2,42	3	0,801
	16	I prevent unwanted pregnancies, especially in adolescents, in the child health surveillance consultation	1,93	2,00	1	1,08	2,20	2,00	2	0,910
	Total F2- Tertiary prevention		**2,35**				**2,42**			
FATOR 3	1	I identify families at risk early on	2,87	3,00	3	0,76	2,75	3,00	3	0,679
	17	I identify situations of domestic violence	3,02	3,00	3	0,86	3,02	3,00	3	0,770
	18	Refer parents with addictions (e.g. alcohol, drugs) to mental health services	3,36	3,00	3	1,16	3,02	3,00	3	1,017
	19	I refer families at risk to psychological support	2,92	3,00	3	1,09	2,83	3,00	3	0,941

		resources								
	Total F3- Early intervention for children and families at risk		**3,04**				**2,90**			
F A T 0 R 4	20	Increasing the number of health surveillance visits for children at risk	2,23	2,00	2	1,10	2,31	2,00	2	0,924
	22	I collect information on social history (e.g. family dynamics, family composition, labour situation, etc.),	2,39	2,00	2	0,98	2,36	2,00	2	0,951
	23	I try to identify the causes of absences from scheduled appointments	2,11	2,00	1	1,07	2,10	2,00	2	1,003
	24	I worry about the lack of information after a hospital stay	2,20	2,00	1	1,09	2,26	2,00	2	1,001
	25	In the clinical interview, I value the family's inability to recall information about their lives	2,72	3,00	2	1,21	2,75	3,00	3	0,679
	Total F4- Intervention with child victims of abuse		**2,33**				**2,36**			

The fact that, in general, the mean, mode and median values are very similar and the standard deviation values are not very high is indicative of the items' good discriminatory capacity.

The internal consistency of the EPCEMtI was analysed using the cronbach's alpha internal consistency coefficient. The values obtained ranged from a minimum of 0.765 (reasonable) for the early intervention in children and families at risk sub-scale to a maximum of 0.937 (excellent) for the total scale (table 5). The categorisation of the internal consistency values was based on the values indicated in Hill (2005). Table 5 shows the overall value of Cronbach's alpha if a particular item were eliminated.

Table 5- Correlation coefficients between the EPCEMtI sub-scales

		Alpha Cronb	No. of items
F1	Promoting child well-being and safety	,849	9
F2	Tertiary prevention	,807	7
F3	Early intervention for children and families at risk	,765	4
F4	Intervention for child victims of abuse	,834	5
Total		,937	25

The correlation coefficients between the EPCEMtI sub-scales (Table 5) are all statistically significant, positive and moderate or high. The highest correlation coefficient occurs between the tertiary prevention subscale and the promoting child well-being and safety subscale (r_ = 0.795).

Table 6- Pearson correlation matrix between the four subscales of the EPCEMtI

		OUR STUDY				CATARINO, 2007			
		F1	F2	F3	F4	F1	F2	F3	F4
F1	Promoting child well-being and safety	1,000				1,000			
F2	Tertiary prevention	,795"	1,000			,675	1,000		
F3	Early intervention for children and families at risk	,679"	,605"	1,000		,566	,628	1,000	
F4	Intervention with abused children	,737"	,708**	,561**	1,000	,688	,661	0,588	1,000

** p< 0,01

Key: F1- **Promoting child wellbeing and safety / F2- Tertiary Prevention/ F3 - Early** Intervention F4- **Intervention with child victims of abuse**

Analysing table 6, we can see that there is a significant positive correlation between the sub-scales, with the value of the correlations ranging from 0.561 for the correlation between the sub-scale Intervention in child victims of maltreatment and Early intervention in children and families at risk, to 0.795 for the correlation between tertiary prevention and promotion of the child's well-being and safety.

A more detailed analysis of the results regarding the practices and behaviours of the nurses participating in our study towards child/adolescent victims of abuse according to the four sub-scales described above (table 4) shows that nurses carry out better practices and behaviours in terms of early intervention with children and families at risk of child abuse (factor 3) (M=3,04) These results corroborate those of Catarino (2007) who found that nurses carried out better practices in terms of early intervention with children and families at risk (M=2.90). Given that most of the nurses in our study work in USFs and that family nurses, in the context of proximity, are professionals who interact with the family system and objectively know the families' needs and, at a macrosystemic level, the resources that the community system can offer, mobilising them to obtain the necessary gains, they can therefore be central to early intervention in families at risk (Figueiredo, 2012, Cit. by Lino, 2012).

In this factor, the item with the highest score for nurses' most favourable practices and behaviours is 18 "I refer parents with addictions to mental health services". Item 1, "I identify families at risk early on", was the item that contributed the least. This is in line with the results obtained by Catarino (2007). It should be noted that 19.8 per cent of nurses stated that they rarely/never identify families at risk early on. A

he early identification of child abuse represents a challenge for nurses, given the difficulty in diagnosing it (Friedlander et al 2006, cited by Catarino, 2007). It is also worrying that 46.5 per cent of nurses reported that they never or rarely refer parents with addictions to mental health services.

According to the OE (2009), nurses are able to identify situations of abuse, refer child victims and promote health from birth to adolescence.

Factor 1 - Promoting the child's well-being and safety, is the one with the lowest values (M=2.15), as mentioned by Catarino (2007). The items that most contributed to nurses' best practices and behaviours towards children and adolescents who have been abused were: "when observing the child, I look for sequelae of the abuse" (M=2.51) and "I value the child's care in different health institutions, emergency and/or permanent care" (M=2.44). These results are similar to the findings of Catarino (2007), although in that study the position of these items was reversed. We agree with the author when she states that "these interventions demonstrate the concern for early detection of abuse situations related to Munchausen's syndrome and situations of recurrence of maltreatment" (Catarino, 2007, p.95) and it is essential that the nursing professional is aware of the signs and is always attentive to suspecting this possibility when it is not declared by the child's carers. In addition, it is necessary to break with the idea that physical aggression is naturalised, i.e. as a legitimate instrument that the family culturally has to discipline the child (Cardoso et al., 2006).

The items that contributed least to the best practices in this sub-scale were: "I assess the quality of the mother/father/child emotional bond" (M=1.93) and "I observe the child's behaviour and the parents' behaviour during consultations" (M=1.75). Catarino (2007) concluded that the item "I value attitudes of distancing, detachment, deprivation of affection and security" (M=2.02) and "I observe the child's conduct and the parents' behaviour at appointments" were the ones that contributed the least (M=1.96). However, it is important for nurses to observe the child's conduct and the parents' behaviour at appointments and the quality of the bond. These interventions are undoubtedly of the utmost importance in detecting situations of child abuse and as the WHO and ISPCAN (2006) state, attachment and assertive parental behaviour are protective factors against child abuse.

According to Silva (2011), nurses should take into account the provision of family-centred care in order to help parents acquire parenting skills. It should be noted that the assessment of the parents' attitude towards setting educational standards and limits for their children was one of the items that contributed most to best practices and behaviours in this sub-scale (M=2.34). According to Bee (1995), the family is responsible for the child's socialisation process and it is through the family that the child acquires behaviours, skills and values that are appropriate and desirable for their culture. In this context, the internalisation of norms and rules will enable the child to perform better socially and acquire autonomy.

In factor 2- Tertiary prevention, the items that most contributed to the nurses' good practices and behaviour were: "I intervene in families at risk in an early, stable and continuous manner" (M=2.96) and "I identify the risk factors associated with child abuse" (M=2.61). These practices and behaviours are in line with those recommended by Magalhães (2005) and the OE (2012), which propose that nursing care should be based on intervention to promote the child's health and well-being. Its absence or alteration can interfere with the child's healthy physical and emotional development, leading to significant health and social problems (Gage, Everett and Bullock, 2006). Catarino (2007) also concluded that the item "I intervene in families at risk in an early, stable and continuous manner" was the highest scoring item in this sub-scale. In the same factor, the items with the lowest scores were: "I value the delay in seeking health care for the child" (M=1.92) and "I prevent unwanted pregnancies, especially in adolescents, at child health appointments" (M=1.93).

Gurgel (2008) points out that in child and adolescent health consultations, nurses have the opportunity and responsibility to identify, deepen and assess adolescents' sexuality and the implications of responsible sex, including early pregnancy. In the same vein, the OE (2010) states that nursing interventions in the context of adolescent care, the promotion of healthy behaviours, both to improve their level of health and to prevent illness, take centre stage.

When nurses recognise the delay in children/adolescents seeking health care, they become aware of the risk of child abuse (DGS, 2011).

With regard to factor 4 - Intervention with child victims of abuse, the items that most contributed to good practices were: "I value, in the clinical interview, the family's inability to recall information about their family life" (M=2.72) and "I gather information about social history" (M=2.39). These results show that during the initial assessment, nurses try to identify and determine situations that may be related to abuse or suspicion of abuse. Data corroborated by Azevedo and Maia (2006), Catarino (2007) and Magalhães (2010). In the same factor, the item with the lowest score was: "I try to identify the causes of absences from scheduled appointments" (M=2.11), indicating situations of neglect of health care, which should be a warning for nurses, as it may be related to other shortcomings, making it difficult for the child/adolescent to fulfil basic health needs (Catarino, 2007).

Agreeing with the recommendations put forward by Fonseca et al (1999), Canha (2003) and Magalhães (2005 cited by Catarino, 2007), who mention the activities carried out by nurses as being of great importance in a child abuse project, we are convinced that nurses still have a long way to go in order to protect child/adolescent victims of abuse.

To this end, a correlation was made between some variables, namely: age, length of professional career, academic qualifications and postgraduate / specialised training.

Table 7 shows that there is a significant correlation between early intervention practices for children and families at risk and the age of the nurses (r= -0.248). The coefficient is negative and weak, which means that the younger the nurses, the better their practices and behaviour towards child abuse. This is contrary to the findings of Catarino's study (2007), which concluded that the older the nurses, the better their practices and behaviours, especially in terms of interventions to promote children's health, well-being and safety.

Table 7 - Pearson's correlation matrix between nurses' practices and behaviour towards child abuse and age

	OUR STUDY	**CATARINO, 2007**
Sub-scales	R	R
Promoting the child's well-being and safety	-,068	,388
Tertiary prevention	,013	,221
Early intervention for children and families at risk	-,248*	-,077
Intervention with abused children	-,075	,185
Total	-,067	,258

* Significant correlation for $p < 0.05$

When we analyse the results in table 8, we see that there are no significant correlations between nurses' practices and behaviours in relation to child abuse and the length of time they have worked in the job and the length of time they have worked in the PHC. These conclusions differ from those of Catarino (2007), who states that there is a correlation between nurses' practices and behaviour in relation to child abuse and length of professional experience.

In relation to the length of professional practice, this correlation is positive for the total scale (r=.209) and for the sub-scales "promotion of the child's well-being and safety" (r=.363), "intervention for child victims of abuse" (r=.135) and "tertiary prevention" (r=.170). With regard to the correlation between nurses' practices and behaviour in relation to child abuse and the length of time they have worked in PHC, this is positive for the total scale (r= 207) and for the sub-scales "promotion of the child's wellbeing and safety" (r=.313), "tertiary prevention" (r=.217) and "intervention with child victims of abuse" (r=.063).

Table 8 - Pearson correlation matrix between nurses' practices and behaviours in relation to child abuse and the length of time they have worked in the position and in PHC

	OUR STUDY		CATARINO, 2007	
	Length of professional career	Exercise time CSP	Length of professional career	Exercise time CSP
Promoting the child's well-being and safety	,072	-,020	,363	,313
Tertiary prevention	,014	,038	,170	,217
Early intervention for children and families at risk	-,118	-,180	-,131	-,017
Intervention with abused children	,030	-,035	,135	,063
Total	-,037	,014	,209	,207

To check the correlation between academic qualifications and nurses' practices and behaviours (table 9), we used only two groups, bachelor's and master's degrees, since the doctorate indicator was not marked and the bachelor's degree indicator represented 5% of the target population. We found the following statistically significant differences:

- Promoting child well-being and safety, t (77)= 2.338, p=0.022, nurses with a bachelor's degree carry out better practices and behaviours in the field of child abuse than nurses with a master's degree (2.23 vs 1.81).

- Tertiary prevention, t (71)=2.956, p=0.004, nurses with a bachelor's degree carry out better practices and behaviours in the field of child abuse than nurses with a master's degree (2.49 vs 1.89).
- Early intervention in children and families at risk, t (77)=2.331, p=0.022, nurses with a bachelor's degree carry out better practices and behaviours in the field of child abuse than nurses with a master's degree (3.17 vs 2.68).
- Overall, t (64)=2.303, p=0.025, nurses with a bachelor's degree carried out better practices and behaviours in the field of child abuse than nurses with a master's degree (2.48 vs 2.03). These results corroborate those obtained by Catarino (2007) who concluded that higher academic qualifications did not imply better nursing practices in relation to child abuse.

Table 9- Results of the Student's t-test on nurses' practices and behaviours in relation to child abuse and academic qualifications.

	LICENCE		MA		TOTAL	
	M	DP	M	DP	t	Sig.
Promoting children's well-being and safety	2,23	0,61	1,81	0,62	2,338	,022*
Tertiary prevention	2,49	0,67	1,89	0,62	2,956	,004*
Early intervention for children and families at risk	3,17	0,70	2,68	0,82	2,331	,022*
Intervention with abused children	2,36	0,83	1,96	0,93	1,623	,109
Total	2,48	0,62	2,03	0,64	2,303	,025*

* $p < 0,05$

The majority of respondents (63.22%; n= 57) had come into contact with child abuse victims during their professional activity (graph 7). This result is similar to other studies (Marcon, Tiradentes and Kato, 2001; Catarino, 2007) in which the majority of respondents had also come into contact with such situations. However, some nurses (12.64%; n=12) didn't answer/didn't know if they had had contact with abused children/adolescents. This result, which we consider to be relevant, may be associated with the difficulty in diagnosing these situations; however, the causes that may be associated with them are not covered in this study

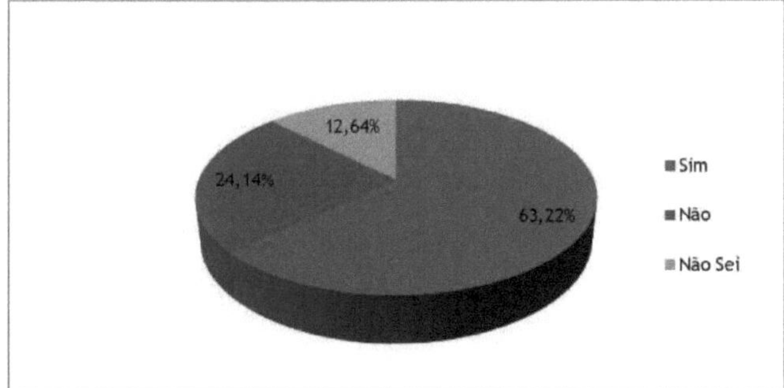

GRAPH 7- Contact with abused children/adolescents

Of the 57 respondents who said they had already had contact with abused children/adolescents (table 10), we found that the situations of danger identified by the highest percentage of nurses were: neglect (76 per cent), parental/family dysfunction (35 per cent), suspected sexual abuse (22 per cent) and physical abuse (21 per cent). These figures are in line with those of the CNPCJR (2012) and Catarino (2007). None of the participants said they had already identified abuse of authority and child labour.

Table 10 also allows us to see the type of action taken by the nurse for each danger situation signalled. Of the behaviours that could be implemented, the most commonly used in the context of professional nursing practice were "refer to social workers" (606), "refer to the family doctor" (576) and "assess/monitor the child's behaviour" (400). Referral to social workers" is in line with the study by Catarino (2007).

It should be emphasised that when they identified a child in a situation of abuse, some nurses didn't act (35). This data contradicts the study by Catarino (2007), who concluded that all nurses took action. This leads us to believe that these professionals do not have the necessary knowledge to refer these cases. This is perhaps a worrying situation if we think that, given their privileged position, they should play an invaluable role in detecting and referring these situations.

This leads us to insist on the need for all nurses who work with children and adolescents to be informed and sensitised to report all suspected cases.

With regard to the most common nursing interventions in relation to the danger situation identified, it can be seen that the most identified were in relation to neglect, the situation was reported (47), in relation to parental/family dysfunction, the nurses referred the child to the family doctor (58) and in relation to suspected sexual abuse, they also referred the child to the family doctor and reported it. As for school drop-outs, they preferred to refer them to social workers. In situations where recurring health problems were recognised, the most common action was referral to the family doctor (63), a result identical to that of Catarino's study (2007). HV was more common in situations of school dropout (40) and neglect (31).

DANGEROUS SITUATIONS	ACTING IN THE FACE OF THE IDENTIFIED DANGER													
	%	1	2	3	4	5	6	7	8	9	10	11	12	13
Abandonment	11	16	16	0	0	0	0	33	16	33	33	33	0	16
Negligence	76	7	26	21	2	29	19	31	24	38	36	47	0	7
School dropout	9	40	40	0	0	0	0	40	20	40	60	40	0	0
School Absenteeism	18	60	60	0	0	0	20	30	40	60	30	20	0	0
Physical abuse	21	25	33	42	0	8	8	17	25	50	42	25	8	8
Psychological abuse	16	22	33	11	0	11	0	0	44	56	44	22	22	0
Sexual Abuse (Suspected)	22	0	17	8	0	0	8	8	8	50	25	50	0	17
Abuse of authority	0	0	0	0	0	0	0	0	0	0	0	0	0	0
Child labour	0	0	0	0	0	0	0	0	0	0	0	0	0	0
Committing a criminal act	4	0	50	0	0	0	50	0	50	0	50	0	0	0
Addictive Behaviours	13	29	57	14	0	14	14	14	14	57	29	0	0	14
Exposure to deviant behaviour models	13	29	29	14	0	14	29	0	43	71	43	43	0	0
Begging	2	0	0	0	0	0	0	0	0	0	100	0	0	0
Recurring health problems	15	25	13	25	13	0	0	0	38	63	38	0	0	13
Parental/family dysfunction	35	16	26	11	0	16	47	16	37	58	26	16	5	5
Other. Which one?	4	0	0	50	0	0	0	0	0	0	50	50	0	0
Total	259	269*	400*	196*	15*	92*	195*	189*	359*	576*	606*	346*	35*	80*

Table 10- Distribution of responses and action in the face of an identified dangerous situation * **Multiple Response**

1-Involve the child to assess the situation
2-Evaluating/monitoring the child's behaviour
3-Assessing/monitoring the child's physical condition
4-Collect evidence for medico-legal assessment
5-Teaching the family about safety measures
6-Teaching the importance of emotional relationships
7- Carry out home visits to monitor the child and family
8- Talk to the parents to check and complete the information
9- Referral to GP
10- Referral to social service technicians
11- Report the situation
12- I didn't act
13- Other. What is it?

With regard to the document used by nurses to report identified dangerous situations (graph 8), it emerged that of the 57 nurses who mentioned having already had contact with this type of situation, one did not name the type of document he used. Of the 56 who responded, the signalling guide was the most commonly used document (42.86%, n=24). The remaining nurses reported on the descriptive report (28.57%, n=16) or another type of document (28.57%, n=16). These figures are in line with those found by Santos (2008) in which the majority of reports are made using a written document.

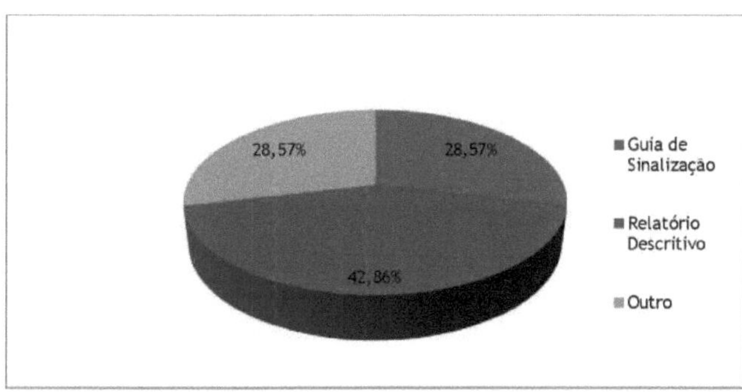

GRAPH 8 - Document used in the complaint

Of the nurses who reported situations of child abuse, the family doctor (67) and the NACJR (62) were the organisations most often mentioned as intermediaries for reporting (chart 11). Fifty-one situations of abuse were reported to the ACES social service (table 11), which states that "intervention should be carried out successively by the entities with competence in matters of children and youth, by the committees for the protection of children and young people at risk and, in the last instance, by the courts" (DL 147/99, p.6117).

TABLE 11 - Organisation to which the complaint was made

ENTITIES	%
Security Forces (PSP/GNR)	2
Another family member	7
Psychologist	7
Social Service Technician	51
Support Centre for Children and Young People at Risk (NACJR)	62
Commission for the Protection of Children and Young People (CPCJ)	13
Family Doctor	67
Emergency services	9
Family and Children's Court	2
Other	4

Regarding the use of a written document (graph 9), either a questionnaire or a risk list, to identify families at risk, we can see that 81.58% (n=74) of the nurses say they are unaware of the existence of these documents in their workplace. On the other hand, 19.42 per cent (n=17) say that they do exist. It should be emphasised that these figures suggest some lack of knowledge about the existence or otherwise of a working tool for identifying families at risk. However, Parton, Thorpe and Wattam (1997) point out that these tools have become a "central" practice in child protection and are increasingly used in several countries, namely Australia, New Zealand, the United States of America and the United Kingdom.

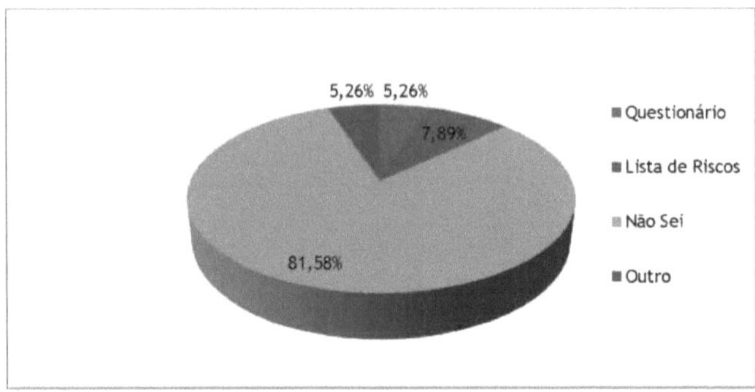

GRAPH 9 - Existence of an identification document for families at risk

With regard to the existence of a manual of procedures for child abuse situations (graph 10), 45.88 per cent (n=42) of the nurses said that there was no such manual in the workplace, 40 per cent (n=36) of the respondents did not know if there was one and only 14.12 per cent (n=13) said that there was a manual of procedures for child abuse situations. These findings are identical to those of Catarino (2007).

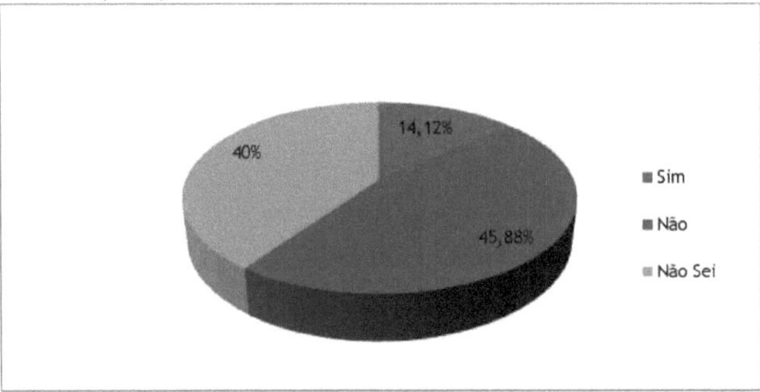

GRAPH 10 - Existence of a manual of procedures for child abuse situations

The lack of procedural manuals for this type of situation is worrying because the DGS (2011) considers them to be a useful working tool for all professionals and teams who, at different levels of care, work to promote the health of children and young people. These manuals have the following objectives:

- sensitise and motivate health professionals about their role in preventing and intervening in abuse;
- clarify and standardise the most important basic concepts about abuse (definition, typology, signs, symptoms and indicators);
- facilitate the identification and intervention processes, indicating *when, how* and *who* should

intervene in a given situation;

• promoting co-ordinated action between the various bodies responsible for intervention in this area (DGS, 2011).

When the nurses were asked if they carried out HVs with families at risk (graph 11), 32.56% (n=30) said that they did not. Data corroborated by Catarino (2007).

The HV carried out by nurses on families at risk is extremely important and allows for a more comprehensive knowledge of the entire family dynamic, economic and housing conditions, family resources and support, as well as the different relationships established between the different members (Magalhães, 2005; Cortês, 2001). Nurses can and should assess family dynamics in order to identify problems that interfere with parenting skills and, consequently, put the child/adolescent at risk.

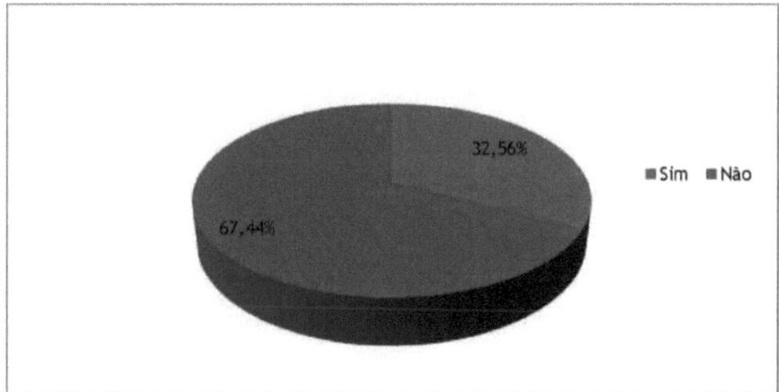

CHART 11 - Home visits to families at risk

Supporting the abusing family can be a positive approach to overcoming situations of child abuse. In these situations, DV plays a key role, because it is the ideal time to develop parenting skills, through moments of EPS, correcting behaviours according to the reality experienced by each family (Cansado, 2008).

HV is one of the activities that form part of the nursing interventions best suited to providing care and assistance to the health of the individual, family and community and should be carried out through a rational process, with defined objectives and based on the principles of efficiency. It can bring innovative results, since it makes it possible to get to know the reality of the child and their family in their own space, as well as strengthening the bonds: user - therapist - professional (DGS, 2002).The nurses who answered that they carry out HV were asked to point out how it contributes to children's wellbeing and safety (chart 12).

TABLE 12- Contribution of the home visit

ANSWERS	**
Increasing the use of prenatal surveillance	33,3
Improving the nutritional status of pregnant women	0
Reduce smoking during pregnancy and with the child	14,8
Reducing parental drug and alcohol abuse	11,1

0 Reduce the number[1] of pregnancies and the spacing between them	7,4
Reduce preterm labour	0
Improving the newborn's birth weight	25,9
Increasing family attachment	59,3
Improving the child's growth and development	81,5
ANSWERS	**
Reducing criminal behaviour by carers	22,2
Increasing the use of health and social services in the community	70,4
Reducing the use of social aid	3,7
Reducing the use of emergency services	29,6
Reducing accidents and poisoning in children	33,3
Providing health education to children	51,9

* Multiple answer

The most popular answers were: "to improve the child's growth and development" (81.5 per cent), "to increase the use of health and social services in the community" (70.4 per cent) and "to increase family attachment" (59.3 per cent).

We believe that the nursing interventions carried out during the HV allow for the detection of situations of proven risk, in accordance with the DGS (2002) Standard Programme of Action in Child and Youth Health, which states that "the assessment of family dynamics and the socio-familial support network should be one of the concerns of the entire health team" (Id, 2002, p.5).) Thus, during the HV, nurses assess aspects of the child's development and behaviour within the family, which can contribute to the early detection of problems and allow them to act on the development of parenting skills in situ, preventing risk situations.

The DGS (2002, cited by Florindo, 2010, p.169) values nursing HV when it states that it expands "the means that enable HV essentially by nurses, as this is a fundamental element of health surveillance and promotion, particularly in the days following discharge from maternity hospital, in situations of prolonged or chronic illness and in cases of families or situations identified as being at risk."

Excellence in care can only be achieved if we get the community, and particularly the family, actively involved. HV is one of the most important activities for ensuring this involvement, helping to improve the quality of life of children, young people and their families.

On the other hand, "improving the pregnant woman's nutritional status" and "reducing preterm labour" were options that were not ticked by the respondents. This contradicts the study by Catarino (2007), in which the most popular answer was to reduce preterm labour.

Studies on the subject (Magalhães, 2005; Rodrigues et al., 2006 Cit. by Catarino, 2007) state that prematurity is one of the child's individual risk factors, making them susceptible to an increased risk of abuse. In this way, all the interventions developed in this area enhance the protective factors, increasing the child's capacity to cope with abuse.

child/adolescent and family resilience according to WHO and ISPCAN (2006) recommendations.

In the nurse's field of action, HPS interventions in the field of child abuse (graph 12) play a central role in promoting health. As such, every nurse is inherently a health educator, since caring is also teaching, one of the components of the educating process.

This dimension is very evident in some conceptions of nursing, such as Leininger's (1984) definition of nursing as "A learned, humanistic art and science that focuses on personalised (individual or group) care behaviours, functions and processes directed towards the promotion and maintenance of health behaviours or the recovery from illness that have physical, psychocultural and social significance for those being cared for" (Leininger, 1984, p.54).

In our study, the majority of nurses (85.06%; n=77) stated that they do not address issues related to child abuse in their EPS (graph 12). Considering that nurses can play an active role in preventing abuse (WHO; ISPCAN, 2006) and that child abuse prevention is centred on health promotion for children/adolescents, families and populations at risk (Magalhães, 2005; Canha, 2003), it seems fair to say that the nurses surveyed need to improve their practices in this area. According to Lima (2006), nursing intervention measures should be aimed at the child's harmonious growth and development, encompassing the family and the community in which the nurse is inserted.

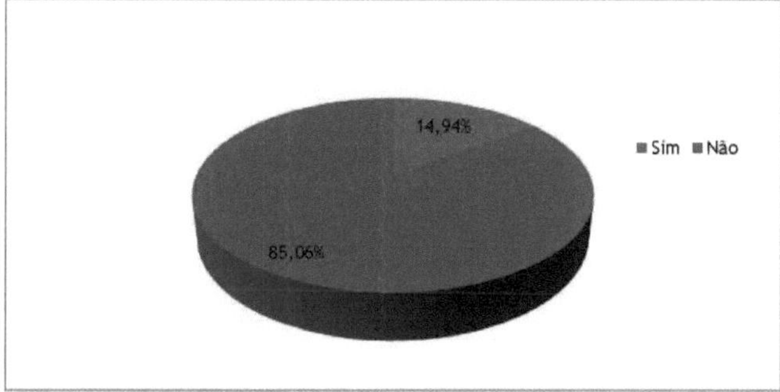

GRAPH 12- EPS in the context of child abuse

An open-ended question was asked to identify the themes developed in the context of child abuse in health education interventions. The answers (table 13) revealed some conclusions, namely that six respondents did not specify the theme addressed, two nurses mentioned abuse prevention, two accident prevention, one sexual abuse, one parental relationship and one neglect. Some of these findings are corroborated by Catarino (2007), the most significant being accident prevention, neglect and eating habits.

TABLE 13 - Themes in the field of child abuse

THEMATICS	INQUIRED
Abuse prevention	2
Accident Prevention	2
Sexual Abuse	1
Parental Relationship	1
Negligence	1
They didn't specify	6
Eating habits	1
TOTAL	14

It should be emphasised that the EPS sessions carried out by nurses are important activities for promoting health and preventing risk situations. For Tones and Tilford (1994, cit. by Fereira, 2002, p.104) a:

> "Health education is any intentional activity leading to learning related to health and illness, producing changes in knowledge and understanding and in ways of thinking. It can influence or clarify values; it can bring about changes in beliefs and attitudes; it can facilitate the acquisition of skills; it can also lead to changes in behaviour and lifestyles."

This definition implicitly and explicitly incorporates many of the factors that influence decision-making. In addition to imparting knowledge, a set of supports will be needed to change attitudes, work on personal convictions, beliefs and individual values (Carvalho, 2001).

As Magalhães (2005) points out, prevention is categorised into three levels:

- Primary, which includes providing services to the general population, in view of the appearance of cases of abuse;
- Secondary, which involves providing services to specific risk groups in order to treat or prevent new cases;
- Tertiary services for victims of abuse to minimise the severity of the consequences and prevent recurrence.

However, these three levels of prevention need to be worked on from an integrated perspective in order to combat the problem. With this in mind, the strategies to be implemented must be based on knowledge of each child/adolescent/family.

In order to identify the context in which they carried out health education, respondents were asked to indicate nursing consultation, school health and HV (table 14). It was concluded that the majority (61.5 per cent) of nurses carried out health education in the context of child health consultations, 46.2 per cent in school health and 15.4 per cent during HV. These findings are identical to those found by Catarino (2007).

Although health does not depend exclusively on the provision of care, but also on a range of environmental, cultural and economic influences, the impact that relevant, quality health education has on the child and adolescent population is undeniable. In a PHC context, the actions carried out by the nurse in the child health nursing consultation aim to provide parents with the knowledge they need to better fulfil their parental role and respond to the immediate needs of the child/adolescent/family.

TABLE 14- Context of health education

LOCAL	%
Nursing consultation	61,5
School health	46,2
Home visits	15,4

3.3- Nurses' training needs

In addition to specific training in this area, nurses working with children/adolescents should also have interpersonal skills and cultural competence (Magalhães, 2005).

In this study, the majority of nurses (88.51%; n=81) had no specific training in the area of child abuse (graph 13), which corroborates the findings of Catarino (2007).

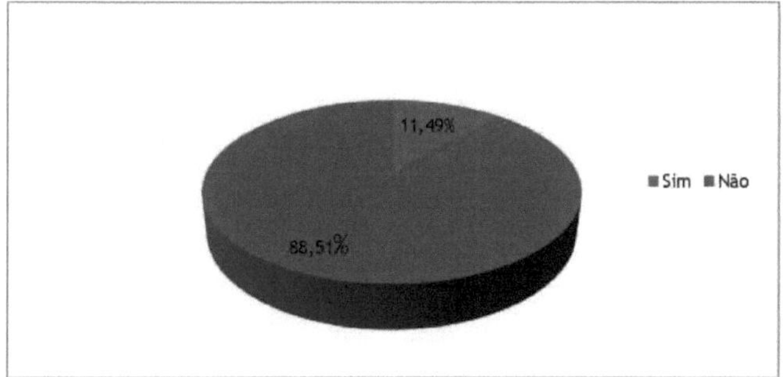

GRAPH 13- Specific training in the area of child abuse

Of the 11.49 per cent (n=10) nurses who reported having specific training in this subject, 8 per cent (n=7) obtained it through self-training (chart 15). Feng and Levine (2005, cited by Catarino, 2007) present similar results, since 87 per cent of the respondents reported not having had any training in child abuse. Analysing these results shows that only a minority of the nurses taking part in the study have invested in specific training on this subject.

TABLE 15- Specific training in the area of child abuse

SPECIFIC TRAINING IN CHILD ABUSE		N°	%
	Formative Moment		
YES	Academic Training	1	1,1
	Training Service	2	2,2
	Self-Training	7	7,7
NO		81	89
TOTAL		91	100

In order to assess nurses' self-perception of their level of knowledge about child abuse (graph 14), a closed question was used in which nurses were asked, on a scale of 1 to 5, to place an X on the option that best corresponded to the level of knowledge about child abuse that they considered they had. Analysing the graph, we can see that the level of knowledge reported by the 91 nurses is between 1 (no knowledge) and 5 (a lot of knowledge), with only 1.14% (n=1) nurse considering that they have a lot of knowledge on the subject. This data validates the need for training on this subject, so that nurses can develop useful and safe interventions. Other researchers (Marcon et al., 2001, Feng and Levine, 2005 and Catarino, 2007) also concluded that some nurses reported having little knowledge of child abuse.

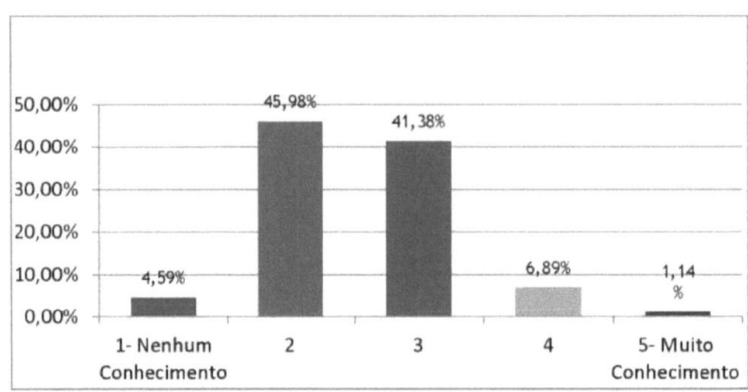

GRAPH 14 - Self-perceived knowledge of child abuse

With regard to interest in obtaining training (graph 15), the respondents indicated, on a scale of 1 to 5, the extent to which they were interested in obtaining more training on the subject of child abuse. Of the 88 nurses who expressed their interest, it ranged from 2 (1.14 %, n=1) to 5 (62.07%, n=55). Data corroborated by Catarino (2007).

These figures are similar to those reported by Marcon et al. (2001, cited by Catarino, 2007) and indicate that the majority of respondents are interested in training in child abuse, not least because no nurse indicated that they were not interested, which leads us to conclude that training in child abuse is an area to invest in.

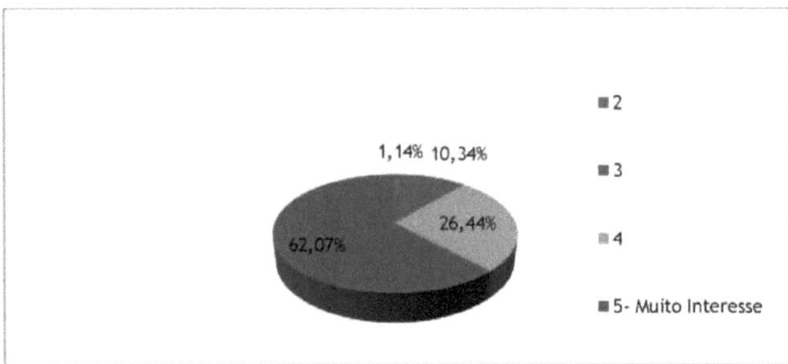

GRAPH 15 - Interest in training on the subject

Of the 88 nurses who showed an interest in training (table 16), the most selected contents were: diagnosis of child abuse (87.4%), family intervention programme (79.3%) and legal framework for child protection (62.1%). These figures are similar to those obtained by Catarino (2007).

Training in communication techniques was selected by 54 per cent of the nurses, which makes us reflect on their interest in improving interpersonal relationships and communication skills, as well as enhancing communication attitudes that facilitate the communication process.One nurse suggested another training topic in addition to those proposed, but did not specify it. The training content defined by the respondents is in line with national and international recommendations so that they have the knowledge to intervene in the detection and signalling of abuse and its prevention (Catarino, 2007).

TABLE 16- Training content

CONTENTS	%
Communication techniques	54
Diagnosing child abuse	87,4
Legal framework for child protection	62,1
Family intervention programmes	79,3
School intervention programmes	27,6
Community intervention programmes for at-risk groups	44,8
Other	1,1

CHAPTER 4

FINAL CONSIDERATIONS

Carrying out this research was an opportunity for discovery and a constant challenge in the journey that is now coming to an end, as it was my first job as a principal investigator.

Throughout this work, it has been recognised that abuse in its many forms and many causes has a direct impact on health and is reflected in the social scenario, generating maladjustments that contribute to an increase in other types of violence.

Various studies have shown the magnificence of the problem and justified the need for an intervention based on scientific knowledge. It was therefore our intention to identify nurses' practices, behaviours, knowledge and training needs in relation to child and adolescent victims of child abuse.

Due to the specificity and complexity of dealing with the issue of abuse, it is essential to share the search for knowledge and interdisciplinary action, so that all professionals can better fulfil their permanent role of protecting children and adolescents. This is an ethical and social commitment that nurses must prioritise in order to guarantee the well-being of children and adolescents.

The conclusions of our study show that:

- 57 per cent of nurses have had contact with abused children and the situations

The most commonly identified were neglect, parental/family dysfunction, suspected sexual abuse and physical abuse. Referral to social workers, the family doctor and assessing/monitoring the child's behaviour were the attitudes most often mentioned by nurses;

- 45.88 per cent of the nurses said that there was no procedure manual for the

child abuse situation. On the other hand, 32.56 per cent also say they don't carry out HV with families at risk, despite pointing out that it helps improve the child's growth and development and increases family attachment.

- Only 14.94 per cent of nurses have developed health education interventions related to child abuse. When they did, the sessions took place in the nursing consultation and in school health.
- The majority of nurses said they had no specific training in the area of child abuse, self-training was the most frequently mentioned context for obtaining training on the subject and 62 per cent of nurses said they were very interested in obtaining further training in the area of child abuse.
- A more detailed analysis of the results regarding the practices and behaviours of the nurses participating in our study towards child/adolescent victims of abuse, according to the four subscales, shows that nurses carry out better practices and behaviours in terms of early intervention with children and families at risk (M=3.04). The factor Promoting the child's well-being and safety is the one with the lowest values (M=2.15), contributing little to good practices.

Based on the aspects presented, we can see that there are numerous challenges and possibilities for professionals working with children, adolescents and families involved in situations of abuse. One of them is strengthening the primary protection network, in this case the family, and the secondary network, which involves various professionals and institutions aimed at protecting and guaranteeing the rights of children and adolescents.

The intervention of nurses specialising in child health and paediatrics should focus on providing more complex care for children at risk and their families, emphasising the technical, scientific, human and relational components, with special emphasis on family-centred care and helping families to acquire parenting skills.

The main motivations and results of this study were fundamental, as they made it possible to find a diagnosis of the issue that could help to improve nurses' practice and behaviour and achieve health gains.

We believe that this study has met the initial objectives of "identifying the practices, behaviour and knowledge of nurses towards child and adolescent victims of abuse and the training needs of nurses on child abuse". These were achieved. Understanding the phenomenon in question will make it possible to implement measures to improve the practice of nursing care for these children and their families, with health gains. We suggest, on the one hand, training measures, covering all knowledge on the subject, assessment tools, referral criteria, as well as teamwork with regular meetings with the NACJR, in order to standardise and provide continuity of care.

The results of this study highlight the importance of developing strategies for the ACES and the NACJR to respond appropriately and effectively to the issue of child abuse. These include raising health professionals' awareness of this issue through training, promoting an institutional culture of care for these children/adolescents through the development of a procedure manual, specific intervention and referral protocols, ensuring a rapid and integrated response with the collaboration of the different functional units, creating a network of informal (family) and formal (community network) partnerships in the area covered by the ACES in which these children/adolescents are cared for.

We believe that this research has contributed to a better understanding of the phenomenon of child abuse on the part of nurses, as well as helping them to realise how nursing care is being implemented and how it can be improved.

At the end of this study, it is clear that there is still a long way to go before children and adolescents can have their most fundamental rights guaranteed. For future research, we suggest developing other studies related to the practices, behaviours, knowledge and training needs of differentiated care nurses and others, with a view to identifying nursing interventions that promote better practices for these children/adolescents and their families with CSP nurses from other ACES.

One of the steps to consider when choosing a research problem is to assess the feasibility and limitations of the study. Limitations are not an admission of failure, but something that readers of this research should consider when examining the results and conclusions. Despite the methodological rigour, this study had some limitations to consider:

• The time available to carry out this research was limited, taking into account the bibliographical research, data collection and processing, as with more time nurses from other ACES could be included;

- Inexperience with the SPSS statistical programme for data analysis.

Knowing these limitations, coupled with my inexperience in research, this study represented a double challenge, both on a personal and professional level.

A final word for all nurses who work with children/adolescents and their families: changing practices and behaviours is not easy, but this work can make a significant contribution to raising awareness among professionals so that they assume their important role in the face of the magnitude and complexity of abuse against children and adolescents. As Senge et al (1994) point out, every organisation is the product of the way its members think and act. Change the way people think and interact and you can change the world.

CHAPTER 5

BIBLIOGRAPHY

ALBERTO, Isabel - Maltreatment and Trauma in Childhood. Almedina: Coimbra, 2006.

ALGERI, Simone - Intrafamily Violence against Children in the Hospital Context and the Possibilities for Nurse Action. Revista Hospital das Clínicas de Porto Alegre, 2007, year 2, n°27, p. 57-60.

ALMEIDA, Ana Nunes; ANDRÉ, I. M.; ALMEIDA, H. N. - Families and Child Abuse in Portugal: final report. Lisbon: Assembly of the Republic, 2001.

ALMOARQUEG, Sheila Rovinski; JUNGBLUT,I.C.O.-ISSI,H.B.- Working for the Reconstruction of Childhood: The Role of the Paediatric Inpatient Unit Nurse in the Child Protection Programme of the Hospital das Clínicas de Porto Alegre, 1999.

ALVES, José Carlos Moreira - Roman Law. Vol.2 Rio de Janeiro: Forense, 1977.

AMBRÓSIO, Ubiratan - Family Representation in Children Separated from Their Families: A Study of Institutionalised Children. Lisbon Institute of Applied Psychology, 2009. Licence Monograph.

ASSIS, Gisela - Violence against Children and Adolescents: The Major Investment of the Academic Community in the 90s. In: MINAYO M.C.S; SOUZA E.R. organisers. Violence from the Health Perspective: The Infrapolitics of Contemporary Brazil. Rio de Janeiro: Fliocruz, 2003, p.282.

ATKINSON Anthony Barnes; HILLS, J. - Exclusion, Employment and Opportunity. London: Centre for Analysis of Social Exclusion, 1998.

AZEVEDO, Maria do Céu; MAIA, Â. C. - Child Maltreatment. Lisbon: Climepsi, 2006.

BAER, Judith - The Effects of Family Struture and SES on Family Processes in Early Adolescence. *Journal of Adolescence,* n° 22, 1999, p. 341-354.

BARUDY, Jorge - The Invisible Pain of Childhood. An Ecosystemic View of Child Mistreatment. Barcelona: Paidós, 1998.

BEAGLEHOLE, Raquel; BONITA, R.; KJELLSTROM, T. - Basic Epidemiology. Geneva, World Health Organisation, 1993.

BEE, Helen - The *Developing Child* 7ª ed. New York: HarperCollins College Publishers, 1995.

BENTOVIM, Arnon; MILLER, L. B. - Evidence-Based Assessment of Parenting Capacity, Family Relationships and the Wellbeing of the Child in Family Violence, Child Abuse and Neglect: The Introduction and the use of Clinically Developed and Scientifically Evaluated Assessment Tools. In: *XIth ISPCAN European Conference on Child Abuse and Neglect*. Lisbon, 18th - 21st November, 2007.

BERMAN, Helene, HARDESTY, J.; HUMPHREYS, J. - *Children of Abused Women.* HUMPHREYS, Janice; CAMPBEL, J. C. - Family Violence and Nursing Practice. Philadelphia: Lippincott Williams; Wilkins, 2004, p.150-185.

BOWLBY, John - *Maternal Care and Mental Health.* São Paulo: Martins Fontes, 1981.

_ Pathological Mourning and Childhood Mourning. In R. Frankiel *Essential Papers on Object Loss.* New York: University Press, 2002.

BRAZIL - Ministry of Health. Secretaria de Assistência à Saúde-Notificação de Maus-Tratos contra Crianças e Adolescentes por Profissionais de Saúde: Um Passo a Mais na Cidadania em Saúde. Brasília, 2002.

The Impact of Violence on the Health of Children and Adolescents. *Preventing Violence and Promoting a Culture of Peace*. You are the key to tackling this problem. Brasilia, 2009.

BRAZELTON, Thomas Berry - *Becoming a Family: The Growth of Attachment, Before and After Birth.* Lisbon: Terramar, 2000.

BRITO, Irma - Health Promotion in Young People Using Peer Education: Interventions with Nursing Students and Young Nurses. Nursing and the

Citizen. Jornal da Seção Regional do Centro da Ordem dos Enfermeiros, Year 7, N° 19 (June, 2009), p.6-7.

BROFENBRENNER, Urie -*Toward and Experimental Ecology of Human Development. American Psychology,* n° 32, p.513-531, 1977.

Ecological Systems Theory. Annals of Child Development, n° 6, 1989, p.249-287.

_ Ecology of the family as a context for human development research perspectives. Development Psychology, Vol.22, n° 6 (1999), p.723-742.

The Ecology of Human Development: Natural and Planned Experiments. Porto Alegre, Artes Médicas, 1996.

_ The Ecology of Human Development: Natural and Planned Experiments. Porto Alegre: Artes Médicas, 2002.

BYNNER, Jonh - Childhood Risks and Protective Factors in Social Exclusion. *Children and Society*, n° 15, 2011,p. 285-301.

CALHEIROS, Maria Manuela; GARRIDO,M.V.; SANTOS, S.V.- *Crianças em Risco e Perigo: Contextos, Investigação e Intervenção*. Vol 1. Sílabo: Lisbon, 2011.

CANHA, Jeni- *Maltreated Children: The Role of a Reference Person in their Recovery. A* 5-year prospective study, 2ª Ed. Coimbra: Quarteto, 2003.

CANSADO, Teresa. - *Institutionalisation of Children and Young People in Mainland Portugal: the Case of Private Social Solidarity Institutions* [online]. [accessed on 14 May 2013], Available at : URL: http://www.ces.uc.pt/ecadernos/media/documentos/ecadernos2/Teresa%20Cansado.pdf2 008

CARDOSO, Emauela da Silva; SANTANA,J.S.; FERRIANI, M.G.C. - Child and Adolescent Victims of Maltreatment: Information from Nurses at a Public Hospital *Revista Enfermagem UERJ*, Rio de Janeiro, Ano 14, n°4 (Oct-Dec 2006), p.524-530.

CARNEIRO, M.R. - *Children at Risk*. ISCSPL,1997, p. 551-574.

CARMO, Rui do; ALBERTO,I.; GUERRA, P. - O Abuso Sexual de Menores: Uma Conversa *sobre Justiça entre* o *Direito e a Psicologia, 2nd* Ed. Coimbra: Almedina, 2006.

CARVALHO, Amâncio; CARVALHO, G. S. - *Health Education: Concepts, Practices and Training Needs*. Lisbon: Lusociência, 2006.

CARVALHO, Graça Simões - *Literacy and Health Education at the Turn of the Century*, University of Minho (Unpublished), 2001.

CATARINO, Helena- *Maltrato Infantil: Actitudes and Knowledge of Educators*. Badajoz: University of Extremadura, 2009. Doctoral Thesis

Child Maltreatment - Nurses' Practices and Behaviours. Leiria, 2008.Thesis to be presented for appraisal and discussion in public examinations for coordinating professor.

CASEY, James - *History of the Family*. Lisbon: Círculo de Leitores, 1996.

COLIIÈRE, Marie-Francoise - Promoting Life - From the Practice of Women of Virtue to Nursing Care. Lisbon: Lidel, 1989.

COLL, Cesar; PALACIOS,J.; MARQUESI, A. - Psychological Development and Education - Psychology of Education. Vol. 2. Porto Alegre: Artes Médicas, 1996.

NATIONAL COMMISSION FOR THE PROTECTION OF CHILDREN AND YOUNG PEOPLE AT RISK - Typology of Dangerous Situations for Children and Young People. Lisbon: CNPCJR, 2005 [Consulted on 20 December 2012]. Available on the Internet :

http://www.cnpcjr.pt/preview documents.asp .

_ Annual Report on the Evaluation of the Activities of Child Protection Commissions - Youth, Lisbon, 2012.
CPCJ Procedural Activity 1st Half 2013. Lisbon: CNPCJR, 2013.

INTERNATIONAL COUNCIL OF NURSES - ICNP Version 2: International Classification for Nursing Practice From the original ICNP Version 2, INTERNATIONAL CLASSIFICATION

FOR NURSING PRACTICE. Portuguese edition: Ordem dos Enfermeiros, 2011. ISBN: 978-9295094-35-2.

CÔRTES, Majó - *Home Visits* [online]. [Consulted on14 May de2013]. Available at : URL http://marcelacortes.vilabol.uol.com.br/visit domici.htm,2001.

COSTA, Elisa Maria Amorim da; CARBONE, M.H. - *Family Health. A Multidisciplinary Approach.* Rio de Janeiro: Rubio, 2010.

COSTA, Maria Augusta Marques de Almeida - *Teenage Pregnancy from the Nurses' Perspective.* Porto: Abel Salazar Institute of Biomedical Sciences, 2002. Master's Thesis

COSTA, Maria Emília - *New encounters of love - Friendship, Love and Sexuality in Adolescence.* Âmbar: Porto, 1998.

COSTA, Maria Manuela Gonçalves Teixeira da - *A Prática dos Enfermeiros em Educação para a Saúde dos Adolescentes* Porto: Instituto de Ciências Biomédicas de Abel Salazar, 2008.Master's Thesis.

CUNHA, Janice Machado - A atenção de Enfermagem à Criança Vítima de Violência Familiar. Rio de Janeiro: Fernandes Figueira Institute, 2007.

CURITIBA Curitiba Municipal Health Department - *Protocol for the Child and Adolescent Protection Network at Risk of Violence* Revista Atualidades. 3ª Ed. Curitiba, 2008.

DECREE-LAW No. 147/99.D.R.I *Series.* No. 204 (99-09-01), p. 6115-6132.

DECREE-LAW NO. 437/91. Official Gazette *I Series.* N° 257 (1991-11-08), p.5723-5741.

DIAS,I - *Violence in the Family: A Sociological Approach.* Afrontamento: Porto, 2004.

DIREÇÃO GERAL DA SAÚDE - Maltreatment of Children and Young People. *Practical Guide to Approach, Diagnosis and Intervention.* Lisbon: Directorate-General for Health, 2011.

DUNCAN, Greg Jeanne, BROOKS-GUNN, J. - Consequences of Growing Up Poor, Russell Sage Foundation Press, New York, NY, 1997.

ENGLISH, BANGDIWALA,S.; RUNYAN, D. - The Dimensions of Maltreatment: Introduction. *Child, Abuse and Neglect.* n° 29 , p 441-460, 2005.

FELDMAN, Kenneth W.; BROWN, M. - Drowning in Child Fatality Review. In: Case M: *child fatality review:an interdisciplinary guide and photographic reference*, Alexander R, Downs eds, GW Medical publishing , p. 311-318, 2007.

FENG, Jui-Ying; LEVINE, M. - Factors Associated With Nurses' Intention to Report Child Abuse: a National Survey of Taiwanese Nurses. *Child Abuse and Neglect.* Vol 29 , p. 783794, 2005.

FERNANDES, Susana Maria Conde - Tobacco and Alcohol Consumption in Adolescents in the Municipality of Mogadouro. Porto: ESEP, 2012. Master's Thesis in Child Health Nursing and Paediatrics.

FERREIRA, Tereza - *In Defence of the Child. Theory and Psychoanalytic Practice of Childhood.* Lisbon: Assírio e Alvim, 2002.

FERREIRA, Maria Margarida da Silva Reis Santos - *Lifestyles in Adolescence: From Health Needs to Nursing Intervention.* Porto: Abel Salazar Institute of Biomedical Sciences, 2008. PhD Thesis.

Efficacy of Implementation Intentions Intervention on Prevention of Smoking Among Adolescents. *Evidence-Based Nursing*. ISSN: 0104-1169. Vol. 14, p.81-82, 2011.

FILHO, Irineu; PONSE, R., ALMEIDA, S. - *Skinner's, Piaget's, Vygotski's and Wallon's understandings of the human: a* short introduction to the theories and their implications for the school *Revista Psicologia da Educação:* São Paulo, n° 29 (Dec 2009). Available at http://pepsic.bvsalud.org/scielo.php?pid=S1414-69752009000200003&script=sci_arttext.

FONSECA, Maria Rosário [et al] - The Abused Child: A Nursing Perspective. *Nascer e Crescer Magazine.* Vol.8, n°4, p. 251-252, 1999.

FONSECA, António - Antisocial Behaviour and the Family: A Scientific Approach. Almedina: Coimbra, 2002.

_ - Children and Young People at Risk: Analysing Some Current Issues. In Children and Young People at *Risk - From Research to Intervention.* Psychopedagogy Centre of the University of Coimbra: Almedina, 2004, p. 11-37.

FONTES, E.M.; LIRA, M.M.F.L. - Physical Violence against Children and Adolescents. *In* VILELA, L.F. (Coord.) - *Facing Violence in the Public Health Network of the Federal District*. Brasília, 2005.

FORSYTH, Bibsi - Munchausen Syndrome by Proxy. In L. Melvin (Org). *Treatise on Childhood and Adolescent Psychiatry.* Porto Alegre: Artes Médicas. 1995, p.1042-1049.

FORTIN, Marie-Fabienne; CÔTÉ, J.; FILION, F. - *Fundamentals and Stages of the Research Process*. Loures: Lusodidacta, 2009.

FREIXO, Manuel João Vaz - *Scientific Methodology. Fundamentals, Methods and Techniques,*

Instituto Piaget: Lisbon, 2011.

FURTADO, Odair; BOCK,A.M.B.; TEIXEIRA, M.L.T. - *Psychologies: An Introduction to the Study of Psychology.* 13ª Ed. São Paulo: Saraiva, 1999.

GAGE, J.D.; EVERETT, K.D.; BULLOCK, L. - Integrative Review of Parenting in Nursing Research. *Journal of Nursing Scholarship* , p.56-62,2006.

GALLARDO, António José - *Maltreatment of Children.* Porto Editora: Porto, 1994.

GARBARINO, Jossey - *Children and Families in the Social Environment.*2nd Ed. New York: Aldine de Gruyter, 1992.

GARBARINO, Jossey; GUTTMAN, N.; SEELEY, J.W- *The Psychologically Battered Child.* San Francisco, California: Jossey-Bass Publishers, 1986.

GARY, Faye; HUMPHREYS, J. - Nursing Care of Abused Children. In:HUMPHREYS, Janice; CAMPBEL, J. C. - *Family Violence and Nursing Practice.* Philadelphia: Lippincott Williams ; Wilkins, p 252-287, 2004

GASPAR, Teresa - Well-being in Childhood and Adolescence: Factors Linked to Risk and Factors Linked to Protection. In Health and Quality of Life: State of the Art. Porto: Escola Superior de Enfermagem do Porto - Núcleo de Investigação em Saúde e Qualidade de Vida, p.171- 176, 2009.

GIMENO, Amaro - The family. The Challenge of Diversity. Lisbon: Instituto Piaget, 2001.

GONÇALVES, Helena - Childhood and Violence in Brazil. Rio de Janeiro: Faperj /Nau, p.257, 2003.

GURGEL, Maria Glêdes Ibiapibina - Prevention of Teenage Pregnancy. Nursing action from the perspective of health promotion. Ceará: Federal University, 2008. Master's Thesis in Nursing.

HANSON, Shirley May Harmon - Family Health Care Nursing: Theory, Practice and Research. Camarate: Lusociência, 2005.

HENNESSY, D.; GLADIN, L. - The Report on the Evaluation of the WHO Multi-Country Family Health Nurse Pilot Study. WHO: Copenhagen [online], 2006. [Accessed 10 October 2013]. Available at http://www.who.int/en/,2006.

HOCHENBERRY, Marilyn; WILSON, D. WINKELSTEIN, M. L. - Wong Fundamentals of

Paediatric Nursing. 7ª Ed. Rio de Janeiro: Elsevier, 2006.

INSTITUTO DE APOIO À CRIANÇA - SOS Criança Statistical Report. Lisbon: IAC, 2002.

JOBIM e SOUZA, Solange. *Childhood and Language:* Bakhtin, Vygotsky and Benjamin. 6th Ed. São Paulo: Papirus, 2001.

KEMPE, Serie; KEMPE, H. - *Maltreated Children.* Morata: Madrid, 1984.

KEMPE, Ruth; KEMPE, C. - *Child Abuse.* London: Fontana, 1978.

KULIK, Eduardo; FLEITER, M.; BATISTA, R. - Nurse intervention in intrafamily violence against children and adolescents. Coren: PR, 2011.

LEANDRO, António de Lemos - Law and Rights: Towards a Real Fulfillment of the Rights of the Child and the Family. Stress and Violence in Children and Young People. Editor João Gomes. University Paediatrics Clinic. Department of Medical Education, 1999.

LEININGER, Madeleine - Care: The Essence of Nursing and Health. New York: Charles B. Slack, 1984.

LEVY, Manuel; CARVALHO, M.C; RODRIGUES, C.C; SANTOS, H.M. - The Abused Child. Lisbon: Portuguese Paediatric Society, 1986.

LIDCHI, Victoria - Maltreatment and the Protection of Children and Adolescents: An Ecosystemic Vision. Noos Institute: Rio de Janeiro, 2010.

LIMA, G.T. - Nurses' records on monitoring growth and development: a focus on childcare consultations. Paraíba, 2009.

LIMA, Licínia - *Child Maltreatment.* [online]. [Consulted on 15 May 2013]. Available at : URL: http://www.multiculturas.com/textos/maustratos children Licinia-Lima.pdf.

LINO, S.C.A. - *Conjugal Violence in Women: Nurses' Practices in Primary Health Care.* Master's Thesis.

LUTHAR, Suniya - *Poverty and Children's Adjustment. Developmental Clinical Psychology and*

Psychiatry Series; Vol. 41. Thousand Oaks, CA: Sage Publications, 1999.

MACHADO, José Pedro - *Etymological Dictionary of the Portuguese Language.* Vol. II. 3ª Ed. Lisbon: Livros Horizonte, 1997.

MACHADO, Carla; GONÇALVES, R.A. - *Violence and Victims of Crime*: Vol 2- Children. Coimbra: Quarteto Editora, 2002.

MAGALHÃES, Teresa. - *Maltreatment of Children and Young People.* 4th Ed. Coimbra: Quarteto Editora, 2005.

Child and Youth Abuse, From Suspicion to Diagnosis. Lisbon: Lidel, 2010.

MARANHÂO, V.F. - Prevalence of child and adolescent abuse in the city of Recife, Pernambuco. Pernambuco: University of Pernambuco, 2005. Master's Thesis.

MARCON, Sónia Silva; TIRADENTES, L.K.; KATO, E.S. - Knowledge, Attitudes and Beliefs of Health Professionals in Maringá regarding Family Violence against Children and Adolescents. *Family, Health and Development.* Vol 13, n°1, p. 35-47, 2001.

MARSLAND, Louise - Child Protection: The Interagency Approach. *Nurs. Stand,* Vol. 8 , n°. 33, p. 25-28, 1994.

MARTINET, Sindy - *Maltreatment: First Signs* - Risk Factors (Supplement 1 - Maltreatment: aggressors and victims in the social context). Inuaf Studia, Year 1 , p.67-77, 2007.

MARTINEZ ROIG, Antonio; PAUL O.J. - *Mistreatment and Abandonment in Childhood,* Barcelona: Martinez Roca, 1993.

MARTINS, Carla - Manual de Análise de Dados Quantitativos com Recurso ao IBM SPSS. Knowing how to Decide, Do, Interpret and Write. Braga: Psiquilíbrios, 2011.

MARTINS, Edna; SZYMANSKI, H. - A Abordagem *Ecológica de Urie Bronfenbrenner em* Estudos *com Famílias:* Estudos e Pesquisas em Psicologia, UERJ: RJ, Ano 4.n°. 1, 2004.

MARTINS, Paula Cristina - *Protection of Children and Young People on Risk Itineraries: Social Representations, Modes and Spaces.* Braga: University of Minho, 2004. PhD Thesis.

MATOS, Raquel; FIGUEIREDO, B - Child Maltreatment: Risk Factors and Protective Factors. *Clinical Psychiatry.* Coimbra. Vol 22, (Jul-Sep), n° 3, p.280, 2001.

Maltreatment and Neglect of Children: Resituation of a Problem. *Infância e Juventude.* Lisbon, n° 1 (Jan-Mar), p.121-134, 1997.

MCLOYD, Vonnie - Socioeconomic disadvantage and child development. *American Psychologist,* n° 53 , p.185-204, 1998.

MELO, Maria Aparecida - Conceptions of Adolescence in Jean Piaget https://artigos.psicologado.com/psicologia-geral/desenvolvimento-humano/concepcoes- de-adolescencia-em-jean-piaget,2009.

MILLER, Brent; FOX, G. - Theories of Adolescent's Heterosexual Behaviour. *Journal of adolescent research.* N° 2 , p.269.282, 1987.

MILLER-PERRIN, Cindy; PERRIN, R. - *Child Maltreatment: an Introduction.* Thousand Oaks: Sage, 1999.

MILNER, Jonh S. - Physical Child Abuse Assessment: Perpetrator Evaluation. In: Assessing *Dangerousness. Violence by Sexual Offenders, Batterers, and Child Abuse*, California: Campbell JC Sage, p. 41-67, 1995.

MINISTÉRIO DA SAÚDE- PLANO NACIONAL DE SAÚDE 2011-2016 - *Estratégias para a Saúde, III.*1) Eixos Estratégicos- Cidadania em Saúde (Versão Discussão). [Online] 2011 [Consulted 10 Oct 2013].Available at URL: http://www.acs/pt.min-saude.pt/pns2011-2016/files/20.

MOSQUERA, Juan José Mourino, STOBAUS, C.D. - *Health Education: A Challenge for a Changing Society.* 2ª Ed. Porto Alegre: DC. Luzatto, 1984.

MUELLER, Nelson; SILVERMAN, N. - Peer Relations in Maltrated Children. In: Cicchetti. V; V. Carlson (eds.), *Child maltreatment: Theory and Research on the Causes and Consequences of Child Abuse and Neglect.* New York: Cambridge University Press, p.529- 578, 1989.

MYERS, Jonh E. B.;BERLINER,L.;BRIERE,J.;HENDRIX,C.T.;JENNY,C. ; REID,T.A- *The APSAC handbook on child maltreatment.* C.A: Sage Publications, 2002.

NUNES, Lucília - *Ethics in Nursing Research. Fundamentals and Horizons.* Loures: Lusociência, 2005.

NUNES, Sónia- *Indicators of Child Maltreatment: An Exploratory Study of 1st Cycle Children in the Municipality of* Olhão-Algarve: University of Algarve, 2009. Master's Thesis in Psychology.

OLIVEIRA, Teresa - Tese de Dissertação: Recomendação para a elaboração e estruturação de trabalhos científicos. Lisbon: RH, 2002.

ORDEM DOS ENFERMEIROS - Código Deontológico dos Enfermeiros [online]. 2009. [Available URL:http://www.ordmenfermeiros.pt/legislação/Documentos/legislaçãoOE/CódigoDeontológico.pdf.

_ Nursing Research - Taking a Stand. [Online] April 2006 [Consult. 30/01/2013]. Available at : http://www.ordemenfermeiros.pt/tomadasposicao/Documents/TomadaPosicao 26Apr2006 .pdf.

Regulation of the Specific Competences of the Nurse Specialising in Child and Youth Health Nursing. Lisbon, 2010.

_ Statistical Data, 2000 - 2012, 2012.

OLIVEIRA, António Manuel Gouveia de - Biostatistics, Epidemiology and Research, Theories and Applications. Lisbon: Lidel, 2009.

OUTEIRAL, José - Adolescer: Estudos sobre a Adolescência. Porto Alegre: Artes Médicas, 1994.

PARKER, Barbara- Abuse During Pregnancy. In *Family Violence and Nursing Practice.* Philadelphia: Lippincottn Williams ;Wilkins, p. 77-96, 2004.

PARTON, Nigel; THORPE, D.; WATTAM, C. *Child Protection: Risk and the Moral Order* MacMillan Press: Basingstoke, 1997.

PAUL, Joaquim de; ARRUABARRENA, M. - *Maltrato a los Ninos en la Familia.* Madrid: Pirãmide, p.13-101, 1997.

PEIXOTO, Ana Patrícia Rodrigues - *Maltreatment in Childhood: A Perspective from the Hill Neighbourhood.* Porto: Universidade Portucalense, 2007. Master's Thesis.

PENHA, Maria Teresa - *Children at Risk.* Lisbon, 1996.

PEREIRA, Alexandre - SPSS Practical User Guide: Data Analysis for *Social* Sciences *and Psychology.* 7ª Ed. Lisbon: Sílabo, 2008.

PIAGET, Jean and INHELDER, B. - *From the Logic of the Child to the Logic of the Adolescent.* São Paulo: Ed. Pioneira, 1976.

PIAGET, Jean - *The construction of reality in the child.* 3rd Ed. São Paulo: Ática, 2003.

PINTO, Teresa; PIEDADE, A.; PINTO, P. - Health Education. In *Saúde e Qualidade de Vida em Análise .IV Congresso Saúde e Qualidade de Vida: Livro de Atas.* Porto: Escola Superior de Enfermagem do Porto - Núcleo de Investigação em Saúde e Qualidade de Vida, 2009.

PORTUGAL. Directorate-General for Health - Programme - Type of action. Lisbon, Maternal, Child and Adolescent Health Division. Child and Youth Health, 2002.

Maltreatment of Children and Young People. Practical Guide to Approach, Diagnosis and Intervention. Health Action for Children and Young People, 2011.

_ *Saúde Infantil e Juvenil: Programa Tipo de Atuação.* 2nd Ed. Lisbon: DGS, 2002.

POLIT, Denise; BECK, C.T.; HUNGLER, B.P. - *Fundamentals of Nursing Research: Methods, Evaluation and Utilisation.* 5th Ed. Porto Alegre: Artmed, 2004.

PRILLELTENSKY, Isaac; NELSON, G. - Promoting Child and Family Wellness: Priorities for Psychological and Social Interventions. *Journal of Community and Applied Social Psychology*, n°10, p. 85-105, 2000.

QUIVY, Raymond; CAMPENHOUDT, L. - *Manual de Investigação em Ciências Sociais.* Lisbon: Gradiva, 2008.

RAMOS, Marta Lúcia Cabreira Ortiz; SILVA, A.L. - Estudo sobre Violência Doméstica contra a Criança em Unidades Básicas de Saúde do Município de São Paulo [Online]. Brasil. Saúde. São Paulo. Vol 20,n°.1, p.136-146,2011. [Accessed 10 November 2012] Available at URL: www.scielo.br/pdf/sausoc/v20n1/16.pdf.

RAMOS, Tânia Catarina - Intervention with Children/Young People at Risk. Porto: University of Porto, 2008. Master's Thesis.

RELVAS, Ana Paula - O Ciclo Vital da Família: Perspectiva Sistémica. 2ª Ed. Porto: Afrontamento, 2000.

REIS, Victor José Oliveira - Crianças e Jovens em Risco- Contributos para a Organização de Critérios de Avaliação de Fatores de Risco. Coimbra: University of Coimbra, 2009. PhD Thesis in Psychology and Educational Sciences.

RIBEIRO, Maria José dos Santos - Being a Family: Construction, Implementation and Evaluation of a Parental Education Programme. Braga: University of Minho, 2003. Master's Thesis.

RIBEIRO, Catarina - A Criança na Justiça- Trajetórias e significificados do Processo Judicial de Crianças Vítimas de Abuso Sexual Intrafamiliar. Coimbra: Almedina, 2009.

RIBEIRO, José - Research Methodology in Psychology and Health. 3rd Ed. Porto: Livpsic Psicologia, 2010.

RODRÍGUEZ LAFUENTE, María Elena - Child Maltreatment. Experiences in Adolescents. Interpsiquis, 2006. [Consulted 23 September 2013]. Available at URL: http://www.psiquiatria.com.

RODRIGUES, Manuel; PEREIRA, A.; BARROSO, T. - Health Education - Pedagogical Training for Health Educators. Coimbra: Formasau, 2005.

SANTOS, Raquel Alexandra Silva - Dos Processos aos Discursos: Uma Análise na CPCJ da Maia. Porto: Fernando Pessoa University, 2008. Master's Thesis.

SARMENTO, Manuel Jacinto - This Child Who Unfolds. In Pátio Educação Infantil, Year 2, n°6, p.14-17, 2005. SBP /Fiocruz /MJ, 2001. Guia de Atuação frente a Maus-Tratos na Infância e na Adolescência. Rio de Janeiro.

SENNA, Sylvia ; DESSEN, Maria - Contributions of Human Development Theories to the Contemporary Conception of Adolescence. Universidade de Brasilia Vol.28 (Jan- Mar) n°. 1, p. 101-108, 2012.

SENGE, Peter [et al.] - The Fifth Discipline. Field Notebook: Strategies for Building a Learning Organisation. Rio de Janeiro: Qualitymark, 1994.

SILVA, Lygia Maria Pereira da; FERRIANI, M.G.C.; SILVA, M.A.L. - Atuação da Enfermagem frente à Violência Sexual contra Crianças e Adolescentes. Brazilian Journal of Nursing. Sep/Oct, p.919-924,2011.

SILVA, Lygia Maria Pereira da - Care for Children and Adolescents in Situations of Sexual Abuse: The Discourse of Health Professionals. Ceará, 2006. Master's Thesis.

SOARES, Natália Fernandes - Children at Risk: Past and Present. Some Contributions to the Historical-Social Understanding of the Problem of Abused and Neglected Children. Infância e Juventude: Lisboa, n° 1 (Jan-Mar), p. 35-51, 1997.

SORIANO FAURA, Francisco Javier - *Promoción del Bueno Trato y Prevención del Maltrato en la Infancia en el Ambito de la Atención Primaria de la Salud.* Madrid: PrevInf (AEpap)/ PAPPS Infancia y Adolescencia, 2005. [Accessed 10 October 2012]. Available at URL: http://www.aepap.org/previnfad/maltrato.html .

SOUSA, Liliana- *Multiproblematic Families.* Coimbra: Quarteto, 2005.

SOUSA, Maria; BAPTISTA, C.- *Como fazer Investigação, Dissertações, Teses e Relatórios, segundo Bolonha.* 2ª Ed. Lisboa: Lidel, 2011.

SOUSA, Arlete; CARVALHO, E.; CORDEIRO, M. - Health Promotion in Child Health. Keeping Children Healthy: Supporting Text 4 (Translation and adaptation of Guidelines for Health Promotion). Lisbon: Direção Geral dos Cuidados de Saúde Primários, Divisão de Saúde Infantil, 1990.

SUDBRACK, Maria de Fátima - *Construindo Redes Sociais: Metodologia* de *Prevenção à Drogadição e à Marginalização de Adolescentes de Famílias* de *Baixa Renda.* São Paulo: Press Grafit, 1996.

SCHERER, Edson Artur; SCHERER,Z.A.P. - The Abused Child: A Literature Review. *Latin American Journal of Nursing.* Vol.8, n° 4, p.22-29, 2000.

SZINOVACZ, Maximiliane - Using Couple data as a Methodological Tool: The case of marital violence. In *Journal of Marriage and the Family*, Vol.44, p.633-644, 1987.

TAVEIRA, Francisco José Monteiro de Paiva - *Analysing Sexual Abuse in Children and Young People in the Intra and Extrafamilial Context.* Porto: University of Porto, 2007. Master's Thesis.

TONES, Keith; TILFORD,S. - *Health Education. Effectiveness, Efficiency and Equity.* London: Chapman ; Hall, 1994.

UNICEF- *A League Table of Child Maltreatment Deaths in Rich Nations*. Available at URL: http://www.unicef-icdc.org. The United Nations Children's Fund, 2003.

VIEIRA, Margarida - *Being a Nurse: from Compassion to Proficiency*. Lisbon: Universidade Católica Editora Unipessoal, Lda, 2009.

VILELAS, José - *Investigação: O Processo de Construção do Conhecimento.1ª* Ed. Lisboa: Sílabo, 2009.

VITORIA, Paulo dos Santos ; SILVA,S. - *Smoking Prevention Programme for the 3rd Cycle of Basic Education*. Council for the Prevention of Smoking. Lisbon, 2000.

The Influence of Family and School on Adolescent Sexuality. Coimbra: Formasau, 2009.

WEINRAUB, Munio; WOLF, B. - Stressful life events, social supports, and parent-child interactions: Similarities and differences in single and two-parent families. In, *Research on Support for Parents and Infants in the Postnatal Period*. New Jersey: Ablex Press, p. 114135, 1987.

WORLD HEALTH ORGANISATION (WHO), ISPCAN- *Preventing Child Maltreatment: a Guide to Taking Action and Generating Evidence*. Geneva: World Organisation, 2006

._ Good Health Starts with Healthy Behaviour [Online].2011 [Consult. 10 Dec 2012]. Available at http://www.euro.who.int/en/home .

Adolescent Friendly Health Services- an agenda for change. Geneva: WHO, 2002.

_ Preventing Child Maltreatment: A Guide to Taking Action and Generating Evidence. Geneva: WHO Press, 2006.

ANNEXES

ANNEX I - Request for Authorisation to Use the Questionnaire

Pedido de autorização Para a utilização do questionário Mau Trato Infantil

Arlete Araújo
Fernanda Craveiro
Escola Superior de Enfermagem do Porto

Exma Sra Professora Doutora HELENA DA CONCEIÇÃO BORGES PEREIRA CATARINO, frequentamos o 2º ano do mestrado em Enfermagem de Saúde Infantil e Pediatria, na Escola Superior de Enfermagem do Porto. Encontramo-nos a realizar uma dissertação sob a orientação da Professora Doutora Ilda Fernandes, cuja finalidade é *conhecer as barreiras dos enfermeiros perante crianças e jovens vítimas de abuso.*

Tendo tomado contato com o trabalho "**Mau trato infantil** - práticas e comportamentos dos enfermeiros", no âmbito da sua dissertação para professor coordenador, vimos por este meio e através da sua pessoa, solicitar autorização para utilizar o questionário aos enfermeiros de cuidados de saúde primários e hospitalares, com algumas atualizações.

Agradecemos desde já toda a cooperação prestada a este respeito, importante para a realização deste estudo que, com boas perspectivas, irá, de certo, irradiar alguma luz sobre esta temática.

Para o esclarecimento de quaisquer dúvidas, estaremos ao dispor através dos telemóveis 96 6352352 / 968431873 . do correio electrónico arl.m.araujo@gmail.com e fernandacraveiro@hotmail.com

Atenciosamente.

Porto, 6 de Novembro de 2012

Fernanda Craveiro

Arlete Araújo

Tomei conhecimento do Projecto de investigação e autorizo a utilização do instrumento de colheita de dados, agradecendo o conhecimento dos resultados.

Helena Catarino

ANNEX II - Authorisation from the Executive Director of the Health Centre Grouping of Greater Porto VII - Gaia

Fernanda Craveiro de Carvalho dos Santos
968431873
fernandacraveiro@hotmail.com

Exma Presidente do Conselho Executivo
ACES Grande Porto VII-Gaia
Dra Isabel Chaves e Castro
Rua D.Maria Costa Bsto,s/n
4430-381- VNG

ASSUNTO: Aplicação de Questionário

Enfermeira a desempenhar funções na equipa de Saúde Escolar da UCSP Barão do Corvo, a desenvolver um trabalho de investigação, na Escola Superior de Enfermagem do Porto, intitulado " **Atitude dos Enfermeiros de Cuidados de Saúde Primários face á Criança e Adolescente vítima de abuso.**"Este estudo tem com objetivos, identificar as práticas e comportamentos dos enfermeiros perante crianças e adolescentes vítimas de abuso, bem como as necessidades formativas nesta área.

Pretende-se contribuir para a excelência dos cuidados de enfermagem, impedindo a perpetuação das situações de abuso.

Neste sentido, vimos por este meio, solicitar autorização para proceder a recolha de dados junto dos Enfermeiros de todas as unidades funcionais que Vossa Excelência dirige.

De acordo com os requisitos éticos da investigação, a participação dos Enfermeiros no estudo é voluntária e todos os dados obtidos são confidenciais e anónimos.

Agradecendo desde já a atenção dispensada, encontramo-nos ao dispor para qualquer esclarecimento que considere pertinente, bem como para informar ao ACES dos resultados obtidos no âmbito desta investigação.

Vila Nova de Gaia, 03 de Dezembro de 2012

Pede Deferimento,
Com os melhores cumprimentos.
Fernanda Craveiro

Aces Gaia Sec. CC
rubenp@csoliveiradouro.min-saude.pt
To fernandacraveiro@hotmail.com, acesgaia@csoliveiradouro.min-saude.pt, 'Drª Elvira Pinto', 'Isabel Terças', Isabel Terças CC, 'Maria Elvira Pinto', pcc@csoliveiradouro.min-saude.pt, 'Council Member Nurse Luisa'

From: **Aces Gaia Sec. CC** (rubenp@csoliveiradouro.min-saude.pt)
Submitted: Wednesday, 9 January 2013 17:33:34
To: fernandacraveiro@hotmail.com
Cc: acesgaia@csoliveiradouro.min-saude.pt; 'DraElviraPinto' (melvirapinto78@gmail.com); 'Isabel Terças' (isabeltercas@gmail.com); Isabel Terças CC (itercas@csoliveiradouro.min-saude.pt); 'Maria Elvira Pinto' (elvira@csbcorvo.min-saude.pt); pcc@csoliveiradouro.min-saude.pt; 'Vogal Conselho Enfermeira Luisa' (lrodrigues@csoliveiradouro.min-saude.pt)
2 attachments (total 208.1 KB)

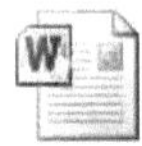

Madam,

Nurse Fernanda Craveiro

On the recommendation of the Executive Director, and in response to the request, the order on the above subject is transcribed below:

"Under the terms of the information from the Clinical Council and taking into account that there is no apparent disrespect for the protection of data relating to users, the study should be authorised. I ask the author in advance for his conclusions and proposals."

Regards

Ruben Pereira

Clinical Council Secretariat Rua D. Maria Costa Basto, s/n

4430- 381 V.N.Gaia Tel.: 227864050 Fax: 227864055

From: fernanda craveiro [mailto:fernandacraveiro@hotmail.com]

Submitted: Monday, 3 December 2012 12:17

To: President of the ACES Clinical Council

Subject: Questionnaire

Good afternoon, Drª Elvira

On the advice of the UAG, the following documentation is available for consideration and subsequent application

I'm also sending a letter to the Executive Director.

Asks for authorisation

Fernanda Craveiro.

ANNEX III - Data Collection Instrument

Fernanda Craveiro de Carvalho dos Santos

CHILD ABUSE

PRACTICES AND BEHAVIOURS

NURSES

Porto
February 2013

Dear Colleague,

I, Fernanda Craveiro de Carvalho dos Santos, am studying for a Master's Degree in Child Health Nursing and Paediatrics and would like to ask you to help me develop a research project on "Children and Adolescents who are victims of abuse".

The questionnaire is anonymous and the answers confidential, which is why we ask you not to identify yourself. Once you have completed the questionnaire, put it in an envelope and give it to the nurse in your unit.

Their contribution is important for the realisation of this research work, the nursing profession and children and adolescents at risk.

Any further information about the research can be obtained by contacting me at femandacraveiro@hotmail.com and/or mobile 968431873.

Thank you very much for your co-operation and availability.

Fernanda Craveiro

Part I: Socio-demographic and professional data

1. Age: ______ years
2. Gender: □ Male □ Female
3. Marital status:

□ Single

□ Married/marital partnership

□ Separated/Divorced

□ Widowed

4. Children: □ No □ Yes

4.1. If yes, number of children ______________ What are their ages (exact years)? _________

5. Academic qualifications:

□ Bachelor's degree or legal equivalent

□ Degree or legal equivalent

□ MasterQual ______________________________

□ DoctorateWhat ____________________________

6. Training:

□ Postgraduate□ Specialised

7. Professional category:

□ Nurse

□ Graduate Nurse

□ Specialist Nurse

□ Head Nurse

8. Place of work:

□ Personalised Healthcare Unit - Headquarters

□ Personalised Healthcare Unit - Extension

□ Family Health Unit

□ Public Health Unit

□ Community Care Unit

□ Pneumological Diagnostic Centre

□ Canidelo Medical Centre

□ Other ______________

9. Time in professional practice: ________ years _____months

10. Time spent working in Primary Health Care: ______________________ years _____ months

Part II - Nurses' Practices and Behaviours in Detecting and Preventing Child Abuse and Promoting Child Welfare and Safety

Read each of the following statements carefully and decide how often you make them.

For each of the items, mark your answer with an **X in** the column that best identifies you.

Answer all the questions based on your usual way of acting. There are no right or wrong answers, only yours.

	Items	Always	Often	Sometimes	A few times	Never
1	I identify families at risk early on					
2	I assess the quality of the mother/father/child emotional bond					
3	I assess the child's care and the presence of symptoms suggestive of abandonment or lack of affection					
4	I assess the attitude of parents towards setting educational standards and limits for their children					
5	I intervene with kindness and empathy, discussing alternative methods of discipline					
6	I promote the adequacy of the parental role and the self-esteem of the parents					
7	I intervene in families at risk at an early, stable and continuous stage					
8	I work as part of a multidisciplinary team to continually assess the progress of the child and					

	family.					
9	I recognise the mismatch between the child's history and injuries as physical abuse					
10	I value the delay in seeking health care for the child					
11	I value the injuries that the child presents at the different stages of development					
12	I value the care of children in different health institutions (e.g. emergency services, and/or permanent care).					
13	I value attitudes of detachment, detachment, deprivation of affection and security					
14	When observing the child, I look for the after-effects of the abuse (e.g. anxiety, social isolation, learning problems, behavioural changes).					
15	I identify the risk factors associated with child abuse					
16	I prevent unwanted pregnancies, especially in adolescents, in the child health surveillance consultation					
17	I identify situations of domestic violence					
18	Refer parents with addictions (e.g. alcohol, drugs) to mental health services					
19	I refer families at risk to psychological support resources					
20	Increasing the number of health surveillance visits for children at risk					
21	I observe the child's conduct and the parents' behaviour at appointments					
22	I collect information on social history (e.g. family dynamics, family composition, labour situation, ...)					
23	I try to identify the causes of absences from scheduled appointments					
24	I worry about the lack of information after a hospital stay					
25	In the clinical interview, I value the family's inability to recall information about their lives					

1. Have you come into contact with abused children during your professional career?

□ Yes□ No□ I don' t know

2. If you have been contacted, indicate which dangerous situations you have identified and how you acted. Select the situation you identified and in the space in front of the situation write the number(s) corresponding to your action (e.g. |x| Abandonment ________________ 11).

□ Abandonment ____________
□ Negligence ______________
Dropping out of school ______________
School absenteeism ______________
□ Physical abuse______________
□ Psychological abuse ______________
□ Sexual abuse (suspected)__________________
Abuse of authority ______________________________
□ Child labour __________________
Committing a criminal act _________________
Addictive Behaviours______________________
□ Exposure to deviant behaviour models
□ Begging____________________
□ Recurring health problems ____________________
□ Parental/Family Dysfunction
□ Other. Which: ______________________________

1. involving the child to assess the situation
2. Assessing/monitoring the child's behaviour
3. Assessing/monitoring the child's physical condition
4. Collect evidence for medico-legal assessment
5. Teaching the family safety measures
6. Teaching the importance of emotional relationships
7. Carry out home visits to child and family counselling
8. Talk to the parents to check and complete the information
9. Refer to family doctor
10. Referral to social service technicians
11. reporting the situation
12 I didn't
13. Other. Which: ___________________________

3. If you have reported any of the situations identified, please indicate the document used?

□ Signposting guide□ Other. What is it?

□ Descriptive report

4. Tick the organisation(s) to which you made the complaint/contact (you can tick more than one option):

□ Security Forces (PSP/GNR)

□ Another family member

□ Psychologist

□ Social Service Technician

□ Support Centre for Children and Young People at Risk (NACJR)

□ Commission for the Protection of Children and Young People (CPCJ)

□ Family Doctor

□ Emergency services

□ Family and Children's Court

□ Other. Which one: ________________________

5. In your workplace, what documents exist to identify families at risk?

□ Questionnaire □ List of Risks □ I don't know □ Other. What is it?

6. Does your workplace have a procedure manual for child abuse situations?

□ Yes□ No□ I don' t know

7. Do you carry out home visits to families at risk? (If you answer **No,** go to question 9)

□ Yes□ No

8. In your opinion, the home visit contributes to: (You can indicate more than one option)

Increasing the use of prenatal surveillance

□ Improve the pregnant woman's nutritional status

Reduce smoking during pregnancy and with the child

Decrease drug and alcohol abuse by parents

Reduce the number of pregnancies and the spacing between them

□ Reduce preterm labour

□ Improve the newborn's birth weight

Increasing family attachment

Improve the child's growth and development

□ Reduce criminal behaviour by carers

Increasing the use of health and social services in the community

Decrease the use of social aid

Reduce the use of emergency services

Reduce accidents and poisoning in children

□ Providing health education to children

9. In the field of health education, do you develop themes related to child abuse?

□ Yes □ No

10. If yes, which topics do you cover most often? ______________________________

11. And in what context? (You can indicate more than one option)

□ Nursing consultation. Which

School health

□ Home visit

Part III - Training needs of nurses

1. Do you have specific training in the area of child abuse?

□ YES□ NO

2. If yes, in which training context did you do it? (You can indicate more than one option)

□ Academic Training □ Service Training □ Self-Training

3. On a scale of 1 to 5, please indicate your opinion of your knowledge of child abuse (put an X by your choice).

1 (No knowledge)	2	3	4	5 (Very knowledgeable)

4. On a scale of 1 to 5, how interested would you be in obtaining further training in the area of child abuse? (Put an X by your choice).

1 (No interest)	2	3	4	5 (Very interested)

5. Select the content you consider important to cover in the training? (You can indicate more than one option):

□ Communication techniques

□ Diagnosing child abuse

□ Legal framework for child protection

□ Family intervention programmes

□ School intervention programmes

□ Community intervention programmes for at-risk groups

□ Other. Which ______________________________

Thank you very much for your availability and participation

Fernanda Craveiro

ANNEX IV- INFORMED CONSENT INFORMED CONSENT FORM

"NURSES' PRACTICES AND BEHAVIOURS TOWARDS CHILDREN AND

ADOLESCENT VICTIMS OF ABUSE"

Researcher: Fernanda Craveiro de Carvalho dos Santos

Nurse at ACES Grande Porto VII-Gaia- UCSP Barão do Corvo
Master's student in Child Health Nursing and Paediatrics at the Porto School of Nursing

I, the undersigned, ______________________________ accept to take part in the research work on the topic "Nurses' practices and behaviour towards child and adolescent victims of abuse", taking into account the following items, about which I have been informed:

- I have been informed that the above-mentioned research study aims to identify the practices, behaviours and knowledge of nurses towards child and adolescent victims of abuse.
- I know that a questionnaire is planned for this study,
- I have been assured that all data relating to identification in this study is anonymous and confidential.
- I know that I can refuse to take part in the study without any kind of penalty.
- I freely agree to take part in the above-mentioned study and also authorise the dissemination of the results obtained in the scientific environment.
-

Name of study participant

DateSignature

_______ ___/___/ ______________________

Name of Principal Investigator

DateSignature

_______ ___/___/ ______________________

ANNEX V - SOCIO-DEMOGRAPHIC AND PROFESSIONAL CHARACTERISATION

Socio-demographic and Professional Characterisation

ATTRIBUTES		N	%
Gender	Male	13	13,95
	Female	78	86,05
	Total	**91**	**100**
Marital status	Single	26	29,07
	Married/married by marriage	55	60,47
	Separated/Divorced	9	9,30
	Widowed	1	1,16
Existence of children	Yes	58	63,22
	No	33	36,78
	Total	**91**	**100**
	Bachelor's degree or legal equivalent	5	5,747
	Degree or legal equivalent	70	77,01

		N	%
Academic qualifications	Master	16	17,24
	Doctoral Programme	0	0,00
	Total	**91**	**100**
Master	Community Health Nursing	10	10,98
	Palliative Care	1	1,09
	Nursing Sciences	2	2,19
	Medical Informatics	1	1,09
	Gerontology	1	1,09
	Wounds	1	1,09
	Total	**16**	**17,5**
Training	Postgraduate	15	16,09
	Specialised	27	29,89
	No Reply	49	54,02
	Total	**91**	**100**
Professional Category	Nurse	41	44,83
	Graduate nurse	40 10	43,68
	Nurse specialist	0	11,49 0,00
	Head nurse		
	Total	**91**	**100**
Place of work	UCSP- Headquarters	22	23,53
	UCSP extension	5	5,882
	Family Health Unit	50	55,29
	Community Care Unit	9	9,412
	Public Health Unit	1	1,176
	Pneumological Diagnostic Centre	1	1,176
	Canidelo Medical Centre	3	3,529
	Total	**91**	**100**

ATTRIBUTES		N	X min	X max	M	DP
Age		91	22	65	36,92	9,12
Children's ages	1° Filho	57	1	36	9,76	8,840
	2° Filho	22	1	20	11,26	8,392
	3° Son	7	1	10	6,29	5,936
Time spent in professional practice Time spent in		91	1	40	13,85	8,701
CSP		91	1	35	8,54	6,607

Item homogeneity statistics and internal consistency coefficients (Cronbach's alpha) of the EPCEMtI scale (N=91)

N° Item		**R without item**	**Alpha without the item**
1	I identify families at risk early on	,354	,937
2	I assess the quality of the mother/father/child emotional bond	,592	,934
3	I assess the child's care and the presence of symptoms suggestive of abandonment or lack of affection	,466	,936
4	I assess the attitude of parents towards setting educational standards and limits for their children	,555	,935
5	I intervene with kindness and empathy, discussing alternative methods of discipline	,580	,935
6	I promote the adequacy of the parental role and the self-esteem of parents	,593	,934
7	I intervene in families at risk at an early, stable and continuous stage	,649	,934
8	I work as part of a multidisciplinary team to continuously assess the progress of the child and family.	,527	,935
9	I recognise the mismatch between the child's history and injuries as physical abuse	,499	,936
10	I value the delay in seeking health care for the child	,436	,936
11	I value the injuries that the child presents at the different stages of development	,655	,933

12	I value the child's care in different health institutions (emergency, and/or permanent care)	,612	,934
13	I value attitudes of detachment, detachment, deprivation of affection and security	,667	,934
14	When observing the child, I look for the after-effects of the abuse (e.g. anxiety, social isolation, learning problems, behavioural changes).	,643	,934
15	I identify the risk factors associated with child abuse	,656	,934
16	I prevent unwanted pregnancies, especially in adolescents, in the child health surveillance consultation	,559	,935
17	I identify situations of domestic violence	,635	,934
18	I refer parents with addictions (e.g. alcohol, drugs) to mental health services	,573	,935
19	I refer families at risk to psychological support resources	,665	,933
20	Increasing the number of health surveillance visits for children at risk	,567	,935
21	I observe the child's conduct and the parents' behaviour at appointments	,644	,934
22	I collect information on social history (e.g. family dynamics, family composition, labour situation).	,627	,934
23	I try to identify the causes of absences from scheduled appointments	,700	,933
24	I worry about the lack of information after a hospital stay	,710	,933
25	In the clinical interview, I value the family's inability to recall information about their lives	,631	,934

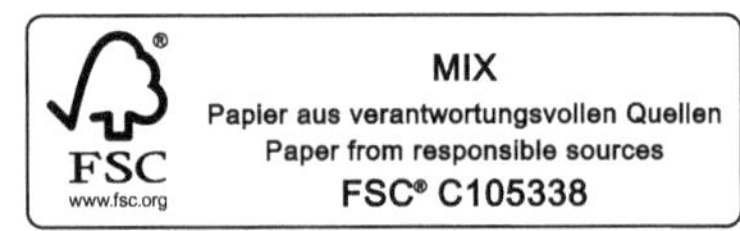

Printed by Books on Demand GmbH, Norderstedt / Germany